SELF-NEGLECT

LEARNING FROM LIFE

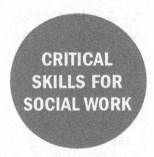

CRITICAL
SKILLS FOR
SOCIAL WORK

Other books you may be interested in:

Self-neglect: A Practical Approach to Risks and Strengths Assessment
by Shona Britten and Karen Whitby   ISBN 978-1-912096-86-2

The Social Worker's Guide to the Care Act
by Pete Feldon   ISBN 978-1-911106-68-5

Working with Family Carers
by Valerie Gant   ISBN 978-1-912096-97-8

Titles are also available in a range of electronic formats. To order please go to our website www.criticalpublishing.com or contact our distributor NBN International, telephone 01752 202301 or email orders@nbninternational.com

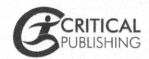
CRITICAL
PUBLISHING

SELF-NEGLECT

LEARNING FROM LIFE

Shona Britten and Karen Whitby

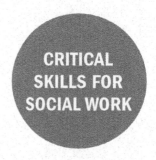
CRITICAL
SKILLS FOR
SOCIAL WORK

First published in 2021 by Critical Publishing Ltd

British Library Cataloguing in Publication Data
A CIP record for this book is available from the British Library

ISBN: 978-1-913453-57-2

This book is also available in the following e-book formats:
MOBI ISBN: 978-1-913453-58-9
EPUB ISBN: 978-1-913453-59-6
Adobe e-book ISBN: 978-1-913453-60-2

Cover design by Out of House
Text design by Greensplash Limited
Project management by Newgen Publishing UK

Critical Publishing
3 Connaught Road
St Albans
AL3 5RX

www.criticalpublishing.com

Paper from responsible sources

Contents

Acknowledgements

We would like to express our warmest thanks to our families for their ongoing understanding, tolerance and humour.

This book is dedicated to the late Gwen Tapsell and her partner Tony Briggs, and also to Karen's parents Kieran and Maura Allen.

Finally, we would like to share our absolute gratitude to Di Page for her warmth and guidance throughout our work with Critical Publishing.

Meet the **authors**

Shona began her career in social work with a charity supporting the carers of young adults with learning disabilities. As a qualified social worker, Shona has worked with adults at risk, in both statutory and independent sector settings. She had held a range of posts including multidisciplinary team and area operational management, service planning and development in the areas of social inclusion and community development, and as a regional director. Shona is registered with Social Work England and is currently a professional lead for social work within the NHS.

Karen is a qualified and Social Work England registered social worker, and has worked within the arena of health and social care for more than 25 years. Karen's career in social work has involved managing learning disability, carers and safeguarding adults services. She currently works as a lead professional for safeguarding adults within the NHS.

In 2018, together Shona and Karen wrote *Self-neglect: A Practical Approach to Risks and Strengths Assessment* (Critical Publishing); this text is the result of their ongoing collaboration and commitment to continued professional development.

Why we have written this book

As social work practitioners ourselves, we have worked with all aspects of safeguarding adults from the inception of *No Secrets* through to the starting point of Making Safeguarding Personal (MSP) in 2010. This has now been translated into a fundamental duty and set of key principles, enshrined within the Care Act (2014), for all statutory agencies and practitioners involved in safeguarding adults at risk of abuse or neglect. These MSP principles also apply to partner agencies as members of Safeguarding Adults Boards (SABs) in England.

We do not aim to replicate all of the excellent work and resource developments undertaken by the Department of Health and Social Care, Association of Directors of Adult Social Services (ADASS), Local Government Association (LGA) and other agencies in England and elsewhere. Our purpose is to describe some of the issues and practice-based situations which can arise for practitioners and to adopt a strengths-based Learning from Life approach in the translation of MSP principles to practical implementation. We base the content of this book upon two case scenarios which are outlined in Chapter 1 and referred to throughout the text.

In pursuit of our goal to aid and support frontline practitioners, and the agencies they operate within, this journey from principles to practical implementation uses a suite of clear and concise practice-focused resources which adopt a person-centred, strengths- and relationship-based approach to all conversations, interventions and aspects of practice. These practitioner resources include a range of *SnapShots on...* a selection of relevant topic areas in work with adults at risk through their safeguarding journey, to practice-based tools for practitioners to use in the quality monitoring of their own casework. The principal aim is to enable practitioners to build a basis for reflection upon their practice and casework within a robust framework for professional development. Each chapter is also supported by a range of *Taking It Further* reading and research suggestions which readers may wish to also pursue.

The primary focus of this work is the UK, where our practice is focused; it refers to legislation enacted within this jurisdiction. However, in clear recognition of the multicultural identity of society, the perspectives of Black and Minority Ethnic peoples and the ever-increasing levels of social work practice development within post-colonial (or de-colonialised) states, we hope that it can also prompt further research and practice-focused works to challenge the potential propensity of Eurocentric positions, which, if unchallenged, may lead to the risk of persistence in inadequate, ineffective and unrepresentative exclusivity that perpetuates the frequently cited marginalisation of Indigenous/First Nation peoples globally. This broad scope of suggested relevance extends to states and countries such as Eire, Singapore, India, New Zealand, Australia, Canada and the United States of America, as well as the UK itself and other parts of Europe attracting migrant workers and asylum seekers. In their paper 'Historical Trauma, Race-based Trauma and Resilience', Fast and Collin-Vezina (2010) examine the impacts, some of which remain multigenerational, experienced by Aboriginal, First Nations and American Indian peoples as a result of government assimilation policies and actions. These are of relevance to practice globally: *'Standard notions of functioning and well-being should be continually questioned and modified depending on what goals the person has for themselves'* (Duran and Duran, 1995).

The style of this text is aligned with our previous publication *Self-neglect: A Practical Approach to Risks and Strengths Assessment* (Britten and Whitby, 2018) in that it is designed to meet the practical, day-to-day needs of practitioners and again should be used to dip into, rather than being read from beginning to end as a narrative text.

Each of the chapters, and *SnapShots on...*, can be used as standalone resources to prompt and support reflective practice discussion. In order to ease the reader's navigation of the text, a brief overview of each chapter is given below.

Chapter 1: The origins of Making Safeguarding Personal (MSP): from principles to practice

This chapter summarises the evolution of personalisation in safeguarding adults, up to and including the Care Act (2014), the *Care and Support Statutory Guidance* (Department of Health, 2018) and related legal duties.

In taking a practical approach to MSP, in Learning from Life, we introduce two illustrative case scenarios in this chapter. We expand these case scenarios within each applicable chapter throughout the book as practical examples and aids to the adoption of MSP in daily casework interventions – starting from initial information-gathering conversations and meetings, the completion of risks and strengths assessment activity, through to the creation and implementation of person-centred protection plans.

Chapter 2: Adopting a Making Safeguarding Personal (MSP) strengths-based approach in practice

In supporting practitioners to make their safeguarding work personal, included in this chapter are a range of practice issues for consideration. The key issues highlighted include: the adoption of active listening skills; an awareness of approaches to societal barriers which continue to disempower and disadvantage people; and the employment of respectful professional curiosity in planning informed and personalised interventions. These resources are included to prompt consideration and discussion of person-centred skills and approaches used in practice. Throughout, an emphasis is placed upon the importance of understanding the person's 'story' and life experiences to gauge and plan empathetic approaches which promote autonomy, human rights and control in making safeguarding personal to the individual throughout their safeguarding journey. These factors are raised in relation to the Learning from Life case scenarios in the creation of conversation frameworks, story boards and personalised MSP bubble graphics, which recognise, respect and positively build upon the lived experiences of the two adults concerned.

The *SnapShots on...* practitioner resources included are:

» The Care Act (2014): eligible and non-eligible needs.

» Advocacy in safeguarding and multicultural considerations.

» The Mental Capacity Act (2005) and best interests decision-making.

» Coercion and control.

» Exploitation, 'county lines' and 'cuckooing'.

» Mate crime.

» A chronology in safeguarding adults (with example template).

Chapter 3: Risks and strengths assessment

This chapter discusses the adoption of a risks and strengths approach in safeguarding adults and wider practice. The Learning from Life case scenarios are developed using a practical approach to risks and strengths assessment, key factors and prompts.

Also included is discussion and description of the issue of legal literacy in key areas of legislation and common law in England; the tensions which can exist between the impotence or refusal of some individuals to manage their own personal health, well-being and safety are also raised in relation to their own potential to effect change.

SnapShots on... practice resources, designed to expand upon and summarise some of the factors of relevance to the Learning from Life case scenarios, and as aids to prompt further exploration by practitioners, include topic areas:

» Attachment.

» The 'toxic trio'.

» Adverse childhood experiences (ACE).

Chapter 4: Safeguarding adults protection planning

In this chapter, the Learning from Life case scenarios are built upon to include illustrative safeguarding adults protection plans, with an example 'Safeguarding Adults – S42 Enquiry Outcome Report' template which provides a simple framework designed to enable practitioners to record the approach and actions they have taken to establish the facts of the concern raised, and the outcome of their enquiry.

 SnapShots on… practitioner resources included in this chapter are:

» The well-being principle.

» MSP and multi-agency considerations.

Chapter 5: Safeguarding adults risk management

Aspects of risk management with adults who refuse to engage with vital care and support services and who hold the mental capacity to make their own decisions and have made, and continue to make, decisions that place them at risk of extremely serious injury or death are considered in this chapter.

 SnapShots on… contained in this chapter are:

» Risk aversion.

» Information-sharing.

» Dispute resolution.

» The coroner and reports under Regulation 28.

Chapter 6: Practitioner casework: critical review and evaluation tools

To promote and sustain effective outcome-focused and reflective practice, and to act as a support in establishing an evidence base for their continued professional development, included in this chapter are examples of simple, clear and concise practice-based self/peer evaluation tools for practitioners to use or adapt.

These simple tools are designed to be used by an individual practitioner to review their casework; they can also be used as a framework for peer evaluation, reflective casework discussion and in professional supervision.

 SnapShots on… included in this chapter are:

» Self/peer case recording review.

» MSP Practitioner 'Reflective Practice' Resource.

Taking it further

References

Britten, S and Whitby, K (2018) *Self-neglect: A Practical Approach to Risks and Strengths Assessment*. St Albans: Critical Publishing.

Duran, E and Duran, B (1995) *Native American Postcolonial Psychology*. Albany, NY: State University of New York Press.

Fast, E and Collin-Vezina, D (2010) Historical Trauma, Race-based Trauma and Resilience. *First Peoples Child and Family Review*, 5(1): 126–36. [online] Available at: https://fncaringsociety.com/sites/default/files/online-journal/vol5num1/Fast-Collin-Vezina_pp126.pdf (accessed 21 September 2020).

Home Office (1998) Speaking Up For Justice: Report of the Interdepartmental Working Group on the Treatment of Vulnerable or Intimidated Witnesses in the Criminal Justice System. HM Government Home Office, London UK.

Introduction

This chapter creates an overview of the germination of concepts of person-centredness, which reach back as far as to the teachings of Sigmund Freud. These concepts were also reflected in the works of John Bowlby in the recognition of how early life experiences can impact upon the adult and their adulthood, through to its continuing evolution in Making Safeguarding Personal (MSP) and the strengths-based approach to practice advocated today.

Background and developments

The experiences of vulnerable people, as witnesses in the criminal justice system, formed the basis of the report *Speaking Up for Justice* published by an interdepartmental working group of the UK Government in 1998. This report also recognised that there were concerns about how crimes against vulnerable adults were identified and reported, concerns shared by the then Association of Directors of Social Services.

As an outcome of this initial work, *No Secrets: Guidance on Developing and Implementing Multi-agency Policies and Procedures to Protect Vulnerable Adults from Abuse* (2000) was launched by the Department of Health and the Home Office; it was the first initiative aimed specifically at the protection and safety of vulnerable adults. This guidance framework aimed to establish local multi-agency codes of practice rather than a national statutory policy framework.

The aim should be to create a framework for action within which all responsible agencies work together to ensure a coherent policy for the protection of vulnerable adults at risk of abuse and a consistent and effective response to any circumstances giving ground for concern or formal complaints or expressions of anxiety. The agencies' primary aim should be to prevent abuse where possible but, if the preventive strategy fails, agencies should ensure that robust procedures are in place for dealing with incidents of abuse.

(Home Office, 2000, p 6)

In order to evaluate the effectiveness and impact of *No Secrets*, the Local Government Association (LGA) undertook a *Review of Literature on Safeguarding Adults Supporting 'Vulnerable' People Who Have Experienced Abuse with Difficult Decision Making* (Klèe, 2009). This review highlighted a lack of evidence or common understanding of *what* type of approaches were being utilised in safeguarding adults and *how* people were being positively supported in their journey through adult protective interventions.

In response to their findings, the LGA and the Association of Directors of Adult Social Services (ADASS) published *Making Safeguarding Personal: A Toolkit for Responses* (Ogilvie and Williams, 2010); this resource included a set of practice-focused resources aimed at promoting the concept of person-centred practice seamlessly into the core of all interventions.

The implementation of the Care Act (2014) saw the formalisation of the personalisation agenda, embedding the Making Safeguarding Personal (MSP) practice principles (Figure 1.1) into statute, and the replacement of *No Secrets*.

The safeguarding duties under the Care Act apply to an adult who:

- » has needs for care and support (whether or not the local authority is meeting any of those needs);

- » is experiencing, or at risk of, abuse or neglect;

- » as a result of those care and support needs is unable to protect themselves from either the risk of or the experience of abuse or neglect.

Figure 1.1 The six MSP principles

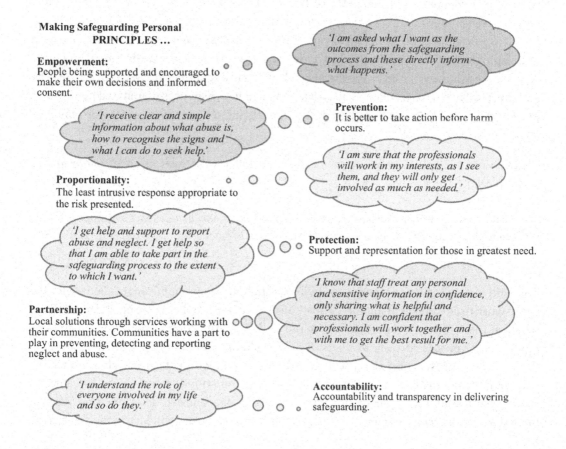

Making Safeguarding Personal
PRINCIPLES ...

Empowerment:
People being supported and encouraged to make their own decisions and informed consent.

'I am asked what I want as the outcomes from the safeguarding process and these directly inform what happens.'

'I receive clear and simple information about what abuse is, how to recognise the signs and what I can do to seek help.'

Prevention:
It is better to take action before harm occurs.

'I am sure that the professionals will work in my interests, as I see them, and they will only get involved as much as needed.'

Proportionality:
The least intrusive response appropriate to the risk presented.

'I get help and support to report abuse and neglect. I get help so that I am able to take part in the safeguarding process to the extent to which I want.'

Protection:
Support and representation for those in greatest need.

'I know that staff treat any personal and sensitive information in confidence, only sharing what is helpful and necessary. I am confident that professionals will work together and with me to get the best result for me.'

Partnership:
Local solutions through services working with their communities. Communities have a part to play in preventing, detecting and reporting neglect and abuse.

'I understand the role of everyone involved in my life and so do they.'

Accountability:
Accountability and transparency in delivering safeguarding.

Chapter 14 of the *Care and Support Statutory Guidance* (Department of Health, 2018) details the legal duties placed upon not only the local authority but also partner agencies such as the NHS and the police. The six statutory principles contained within paragraph 14.13 (empowerment, prevention, proportionality, protection, partnership and accountability) are described in Figure 1.1.

The authors advocate the use of this set of fundamental principles as a guiding framework in all aspects of social work practice, not solely in relation to safeguarding adults casework, and believe they are immensely useful for all jurisdictions to adopt.

Changes to the practitioner role

So, the question arises of how MSP differs from previous statutory social work practices which had been in place since the implementation of the NHS and Community Care Act (1990). Fundamentally, as many readers will recognise, the NHS and Community Care Act introduced, and imposed, significant challenges to values-based social work practice, with a shift of the statutory social work role to one of 'care manager', and as 'commissioner' of care/ support services.

According to a paper published in the *British Journal of Social Work* (Lymbery, 1998), there was no clear blueprint for the change to a care management system. Theories differed as to how it would impact on professional social workers. Some argued that care management as an approach to meeting the needs of older people was both more professional and more co-ordinated; however, concerns were also raised regarding the deskilling of social workers, and the greater emphasis on managerialist and technical responses dominated by resource priorities. Generally it was thought that care management had moved social work towards an administrative model.

This view is echoed in various texts of the time, such as *A Crisis in Care? Challenges to Social Work*:

If social workers are redefined as care managers – as 'purchasers' – then the balance of their professional role seems to shift explicitly to one of management, even if it is 'management' of a rather particular type.

(Clarke, 1993, p 80)

This shift in emphasis, and statutory duty, in our opinion, posed significant challenges for the social work profession to maintain the position of the person at the centre of all interventions when, at the forefront, responsibilities required the identification of solutions which were management process-driven. In the UK, this neoliberal agenda has continued to develop from the years of Thatcherism through to current times; however, the profession, both in the UK and internationally, has continued to thrive based upon fundamental human values of rights, responsibilities, opportunities, independence, safety and self-determination. We promote that the challenge of managerialism has, in fact, developed resilience in the profession, with many practitioners welcoming the implementation of the Care Act (2014) and MSP as a return to 'real' social work.

In the continuing face of a reducing welfare state, and growing social divisions, challenges remain for social workers as skilled navigators within their local communities, in seeking to maintain human values as their core business. Rather than theorising about the potential impacts of MSP, this practice-based text is built upon learning from the people who have, and are continuing to, experience the translation of principles into their life choices.

Learning from Life case scenarios

In both of the case scenarios, briefly outlined below, multi-agency safeguarding adults policy and procedures were followed, and both individuals met the three-stage criteria contained within the *Care and Support Statutory Guidance*:

The safeguarding duties apply to an adult who:

» *has needs for care and support (whether or not the local authority is meeting any of those needs)*

» *is experiencing, or at risk of, abuse or neglect*

» *as a result of those care and support needs is unable to protect themselves from either the risk of, or the experience of abuse or neglect.*

(Department of Health, 2018, para 14.2)

Scenario one – JA

JA is a male in his mid-50s. He lives alone in a privately rented house in a small town; he has lived at this address for nearly ten years. JA has a history of inpatient treatment under Section 3 of the Mental Health Act (1983) and has a diagnosis of '*6A02.0 Autism spectrum disorder without disorder of intellectual development and with mild or no impairment of functional language*' (WHO, 2018).

JA's main source of support is his elderly mother; however, she lives some distance away and her own health has been failing over recent years.

A dispute had arisen between JA and a neighbour; this neighbour contacted the local council to raise concerns that JA's home environment was insanitary. The Environmental Health department has raised a Safeguarding Concern, as on visiting the address they had significant concerns.

Scenario two – CD

CD is a female in her mid-40s. She lives alone in a council flat in an inner-city area; she receives ongoing support to maintain her mental health well-being and responsibilities in relation to her tenancy. CD has a history of mental health problems, including serious self-harming behaviours, and was discharged from hospital a year earlier after an extended stay. The support worker has raised a Safeguarding Concern as she has become concerned that CD may be subject to financial exploitation; CD is aware that concerns have been raised.

The social work theory base

In approaching each of these Learning from Life case scenarios, we openly combined key elements of person-centred theory – empathy, unconditional positive regard and genuineness (Rogers, 1959) – with relationship-based and solution-focused practice in the context of the social model of disability (Oliver, 1983, 1990, 2013). This may appear to be an incongruent mix; however, when used in clear, well-planned and thought-through ways, we suggest that these types of blended theory base are in fact commonly adopted practice.

Social workers can utilize a single theory or method, or they may choose to take an eclectic approach. An eclectic approach involves the social worker selecting different theories and methods and combining all or various aspects of them in practice.

(Teater, 2014, p 6)

We do not intend to analyse the complexity of theory base in social work as this is not linear in form and is often described as eclectic; there are many authoritative texts available. In extremely simple terms, person-centred theory is an approach to psychotherapy practice, originally described by the late Carl Rogers in the mid-twentieth century. Relationship-based practice promotes the person as the source of control, who defines for themself the outcomes/change they want to achieve, with the practitioner as the means by which the person is enabled to self-actualise – the relationship between the person and the practitioner being the vehicle to achievement (this is not an exhaustive description or analysis). In statutory settings the possibility of person-centred theory and practice being the sole intervention base is questionable (Murphy et al, 2013); therefore, in our own practice, we recognise that in building a respectful and enabling relationship to support the person to identify the outcomes they wish to achieve also requires the purpose of conversations and involvement to be clearly and honestly clarified at the start of the process. This clarification process involves the maintenance of a positive focus upon solutions, with the recognition that there may well be time-sensitive tasks or actions to be clarified, agreed and undertaken. In some circumstances the person–practitioner relationship in itself may be the solution to the concerns or risks posed; however, in relation to the Learning from Life case scenarios this was not the case.

A strengths-based approach

With the inception of the Care Act (2014), which guided the taking of a strengths-based approach in practice, further clarity of structure and practitioner resources have been much sought after. The opening paragraphs of the associated *Care and Support Statutory Guidance* detail.

Paragraph 1.1

*The core purpose of adult care and support is to help people to achieve the outcomes that matter to them in their life. Throughout this guidance document, the different chapters set out how a local authority should go about performing its care and support responsibilities. **Underpinning all of these individual 'care and support functions' (that is, any process, activity or broader responsibility that the local authority performs) is the need to ensure that doing so focuses on the needs and goals of the person concerned.***

Paragraph 1.2

Local authorities must promote wellbeing when carrying out any of their care and support functions in respect of a person. This may sometimes be referred to as 'the wellbeing principle' because it is a guiding principle that puts wellbeing at the heart of care and support.

Paragraph 1.3

The wellbeing principle applies in all cases where a local authority is carrying out a care and support function, or making a decision, in relation to a person. For this reason it is referred to throughout this guidance. It applies equally to adults with care and support needs and their carers.

(Department of Health, 2018, emphasis added)

The practice framework and practice handbook published by the Department of Health and Social Care (Baron and Stanley, 2019) provides an extensive resource for all practitioners to utilise in the further development of their knowledge, skill and expertise in the promotion and achievement of personalisation. We actively promote its exploration and use by practitioners from all sectors and agencies involved in promoting the well-being of adults with care and support needs, including safeguarding. The model approach to practice suggested in this work is referred to as KcVETS (Figure 1.2) and is described as

an agreed framework needs to reinforce ideas of up to date practice and co-produced knowledge (Kc) and research, promote our social work values (V) and ethics, render visible social work theories (T) and methods, and promote a range of practice skills (S). The practitioner's experiential learning is also recognised (E) and promoted and this is important if we are to avoid prescription and promote professional judgement and professional decision making.

(Baron and Stanley, 2019, p 3)

Figure 1.2 The KcVETS framework

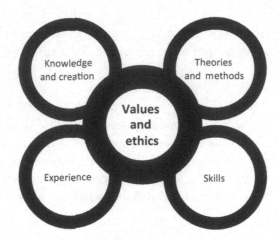

Conclusion

This chapter has taken a short exploratory journey through the evolution of practice to person-centred and personalised safeguarding, embodied in MSP. The Learning from Life case scenarios have also been introduced and will be referred to later in the book. Commentary has also been included regarding changes to the social work role for practitioners in the UK over the past 30 years and the shift from a role of care management to that of a partnership in care and support planning with the values of autonomy, empowerment, rights and social justice as core facets. The chief social worker in England, Lyn Romeo, in the *Knowledge and Skills Statement for Social Workers in Adult Services* published by the Department of Health in March 2015 confirmed that:

Social workers should have a critical understanding of the difference between theory, research, evidence and expertise and the role of professional judgement. They should use practice evidence and research to inform the complex judgements and decisions needed to support, empower and protect their service users. They should apply imagination, creativity and curiosity to working in partnership with individuals and their carers, acknowledging the centrality of people's own expertise about their experience and needs.

(Romeo, 2015, p 5)

Taking it further

References

Baron, S and Stanley, T (2019) *Strengths-based Approach: Practice Framework and Practice Handbook.* London: Department of Health and Social Care. [online] Available at: https://assets.publishing.service.gov.uk/government/uploads/system/uploads/attachment_data/file/778134/stengths-based-approach-practice-framework-and-handbook.pdf (accessed 21 September 2020).

Clarke, E (ed) (1993) *A Crisis in Care? Challenges to Social Work.* London: The Open University and Sage Publications Ltd.

Department of Health (2018) *Care and Support Statutory Guidance*. London: HM Government Department of Health and Social Care. [online] Available at: www.gov.uk/government/publications/care-act-statutory-guidance/care-and-support-statutory-guidance (accessed 21 September 2020).

Home Office (2000) *No Secrets: Guidance on Developing and Implementing Multi-agency Policies and Procedures to Protect Vulnerable Adults from Abuse*. London: HM Government Home Office and Department of Health.

Klèe, D (2009) *Review of Literature on Safeguarding Adults Supporting 'Vulnerable' People Who Have Experienced Abuse with Difficult Decision Making*. London: Local Government Association (LGA).

Lymbery, M (1998) Care Management and Professional Autonomy: The Impact of Community Care Legislation on Social Work with Older People. *British Journal of Social Work*, 28(6): 863–78.

Murphy, D, Duggan, M and Joseph, S (2013) Relationship-Based Social Work and Its Compatibility with the Person-Centred Approach: Principled versus Instrumental Perspectives. *British Journal of Social Work*, 43(4): 703–19. [online] Available at: https://doi.org/10.1093/bjsw/bcs003 (accessed 13 November 2020).

Ogilvie, K and Williams, C (2010) *Making Safeguarding Personal: A Toolkit for Responses*. London: Local Government Association (LGA).

Oliver, M (1983) *Social Work with Disabled People*. Basingstoke: Macmillan.

Oliver, M (1990) *The Politics of Disablement*. Basingstoke: Macmillan.

Oliver, M (2013) The Social Model of Disability: Thirty Years On. *Disability & Society*, 28(7): 1024–26.

Rogers, C (1959) A Theory of Therapy, Personality and Interpersonal Relationships as Developed in the Client-centered Framework. In Koch, S (ed) *Psychology: A Study of a Science, Vol. 3: Formulations of the Person and the Social Context*. New York: McGraw Hill. [online] Available at: https://archive.org/stream/psychologyastudy017916mbp/psychologyastudy017916mbp_djvu.txt (accessed 21 September 2020).

Romeo, L (2015) *Knowledge and Skills Statement for Social Workers in Adult Services*. London: Department of Health. [online] Available at: https://lynromeo.blog.gov.uk/wp-content/uploads/sites/70/2015/03/KSS_for_Social_Workers_in_Adult_Services.pdf (accessed 21 September 2020).

Teater, B (2014) *An Introduction to Applying Social Work Theories and Methods*, 2nd edition. Maidenhead: Open University Press.

World Health Organization (WHO) (2018) *International Classification of Diseases – 11*. [online] Available at: www.who.int/classifications/icd/en/ (accessed 21 September 2020).

Publications

Collins, A (2014) *Measuring What Really Matters*. London: The Health Foundation. [online] Available at: www.health.org.uk/sites/default/files/MeasuringWhatReallyMatters.pdf (accessed 21 September 2020).

Local Government Association and ADASS (2015) *Adult Safeguarding and Domestic Abuse: A Guide to Support Practitioners and Managers*. London: ADASS. [online] Available at: www.local.gov.uk/sites/default/files/documents/adult-safeguarding-and-do-cfe.pdf (accessed 21 September 2020).

Websites

Social Care Institute for Excellence (SCIE) (nd) *Personalisation – Making It Happen: Black and Minority Ethnic (BME) Communities*. [online] Available at: www.scie.org.uk/personalisation/specific-groups/bme (accessed 21 September 2020).

The Health Foundation (2014) *Person-centred care made simple*. [online] Available at: www.basw.co.uk/system/files/resources/basw_25220-6_0.pdf (accessed 21 September 2020).

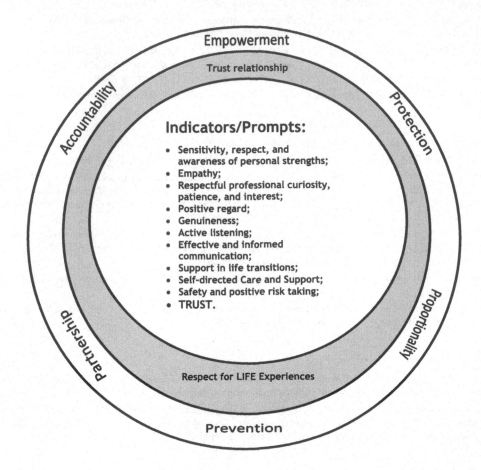

Introduction

As highlighted in Chapter 1, the Care Act (2014) in England and Wales has required a significant shift in thinking and practice regarding the role of social workers and social care practitioners in their involvement with adults with care and support needs. Practitioners retain responsibility for assessment of need and 'well-being' measured against a set of eligibility criteria which are common across all geographic areas. However, the primary focus in MSP is in the adult themselves as the driver of all planning to meet their eligible needs, with the practitioner as an enabler as opposed to them being part of a care management process in the role of lead 'commissioner' of services. A '*SnapShot on... the well-being principle*' can be found in Chapter 4 of this text, with a *'SnapShot on...* eligible and non-eligible needs' included later in this chapter.

In order to efficiently fulfil this role of enabler, practitioners are required to continually build their practice toolkit, knowledge and skill base. This toolkit should include knowledge about the range of support resources available within the local community, as well as developments in practice theory, research and legislation. In this chapter, we aim to raise issues for consideration and key approaches to practice as aids to informed needs assessment and future care/support planning. This includes recognition of significant societal factors, which are discussed further below, and life experiences which may impact upon an adult and their ability to be fully and effectively involved in safeguarding processes.

Taking an enabling approach in contacts with adults with care and support needs is of relevance to all types of practitioner who may be involved; this includes care/support workers, nurses and healthcare professionals in both primary and secondary care settings, police officers, teachers, housing officers, Environmental Health officers as well as those who work in the wider private, voluntary and charity sectors.

Included in this chapter are the following *SnapShot on...* resources:

» The Care Act (2014): eligible and non-eligible needs.

» Advocacy in safeguarding and multicultural considerations.

» The Mental Capacity Act (2005) and best interests decision-making.

» Coercion and control.

» Exploitation, 'county lines' and 'cuckooing'.

» Mate crime.

» A chronology in safeguarding adults (with example template).

Inclusion and empowerment

The adoption and commitment to the achievement of MSP and effective socially and personally inclusive practice requires practitioners to proactively pursue empowerment and equality with people who have care and support needs, recognising that adjustments to the environment and structure of activity may often be required. In the context of safeguarding adults, this includes, when required, the provision of advocacy and/or additional support to the person to enable and empower them to freely identify the self-defined outcomes they wish to achieve, as in all other practice interventions.

In giving meaning to MSP it is important to view practice in the context of anti-discriminatory practice (ADP) and anti-oppressive practice (AOP) approaches to achieve human rights and social justice. The following statement was approved by the International Federation of Social Workers (IFSW) General Meeting and the International Association of Schools of Social Work (IASSW) General Assembly in 2014 as the global definition of the social work profession:

Social work is a practice-based profession and an academic discipline that promotes social change and development, social cohesion, and the empowerment and liberation of people. Principles of social justice, human rights, collective responsibility and respect for diversities are central to social work. Underpinned by theories of social work, social sciences, humanities and indigenous knowledge, social work engages people and structures to address life challenges and enhance wellbeing. The above definition may be amplified at national and/or regional levels.

(IFSW, 2014)

We encourage readers to explore further the principles outlined within the global definition above. To give a practical and accessible view of factors to consider in all interventions, we find what are referred to as 'Models of Disability' as effective resources from which to support recognition of the fundamental equality and human rights of the person, within the context of societal barriers. This is not in any way to ignore or marginalise the vast array of research and published texts about ADP and AOP; more it is a pragmatic starting point from which practitioners can measure and develop their own practice. The medical and social models of disability are briefly described below and should be read in the context of full awareness of wider systemic factors which continue to oppress, discriminate against and marginalise members of society because of, for example, their age, gender, race, cultural identity, sexual orientation, religion and beliefs (not exhaustive or exclusive).

The two most frequently mentioned 'Models of Disability' which have been recognised over the past 30-plus years are the 'medical' and 'social' models; the latter first defined by Professor Michael Oliver in the 1980s (Oliver, 1983).

The 'medical' model of disability

The 'medical' model of disability views disability as a 'problem' or set of problems to be solved, which belong to and are focused upon the individual disabled person themself; it does not recognise discrimination and inequality as systemic societal obstacles and matters of critical political and personal concern. This approach to disability, as the term suggests, is founded upon the individualised approach to clinical and medical practice; we summarise this approach as 'you have the problems and these are the things that we, the professionals, need to do to cure you'.

Our graphic representation (Figure 2.1) shows how the disabled person is the receiver of input and intervention, not the guide or decision-maker of what happens to them.

Figure 2.1 A 'medical' model of disability

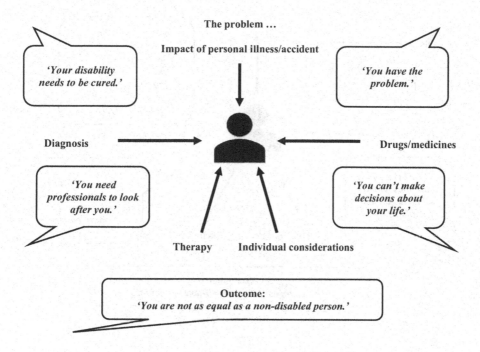

The 'social' model of disability

In complete contrast, the social model of disability places responsibility on society for the mitigation and wherever possible the eradication of obstacles and disabling barriers to the full inclusion and participation of disabled people as citizens, as a fundamental human rights issue. Societal barriers to the full participation and citizenship of disabled people are the matters to be addressed, not solely or in isolation from the person's individual needs. This approach to inclusion places emphasis upon personal and political action taking 'centre space' rather than the issues being subject to societal marginalisation. This sense of marginalisation can be further compounded by other individual characteristics such as age, sex, gender reassignment, sexual orientation, race and religion or belief.

Our graphic representation of this model (Figure 2.2) is designed to reflect the continuing need for society to respect and proactively work to address and eradicate barriers which disable people, and compound exclusion, discrimination and the disempowerment of people who are equal citizens.

Professor Michael Oliver (Emeritus Professor of Disability Studies at the University of Greenwich) first defined the concept of the 'Social Model of Disability' and has written widely on this issue. We strongly recommend practitioners explore the works he has produced; suggested texts are Oliver (1983, 1990, 2013), included in the *Taking It Further* section at the end of this chapter.

Figure 2.2 A 'social' model of disability

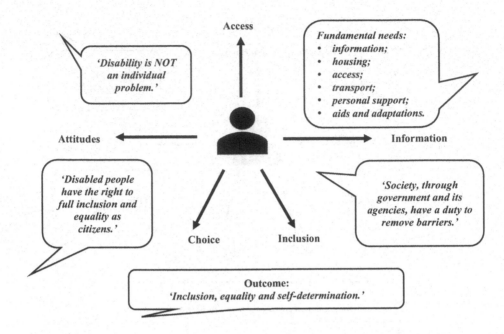

Active listening

Figure 2.3 'Top tips' for active listening

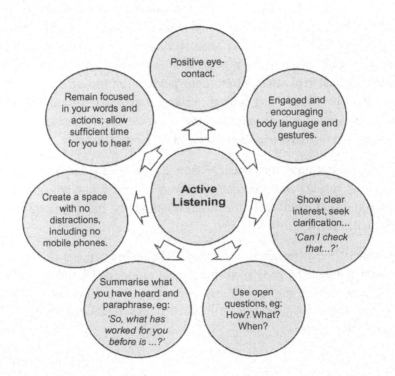

One of the key fundamentals in achieving personalisation in practice is the ability to employ active listening in all practice interventions, as a means to establish and maintain a relationship based upon empathy, unconditional positive regard and genuineness – concepts described by Carl Rogers (1959).

Figure 2.3 outlines some top tips in the development of active listening skills. It is a skill that does need to be learned and continually checked, to ensure that we are demonstrating interest and commitment to the person we are engaged with.

The environment and time

When arranging the meeting, be led by the person. They may feel more comfortable in their own home or in an outside environment (in cases of alleged self-neglect consider if avoidance of issues of concern, such as extreme clutter or an insanitary environment, may be a factor); always ensure that you have allowed sufficient time.

If the meeting is to take place in the person's own home, think about where you place yourself to have a conversation with them. Ask yourself, can I hear them, and can they hear me? Can I see the person; are we facing each other? As the meeting progresses consider if this is the best place to meet or should you suggest meeting away from the home to continue the conversation? This can be of extreme importance in cases where the person says and/or appears concerned that they may be coerced or influenced by others who may come into the room or be listening outside.

If the meeting is to be held away from the person's own home, ensure that the room/space is available for enough time to allow the person to begin to speak and tell their story. Be aware of and take necessary actions to minimise sources of potential distraction and interruption; these can include the lighting (is it too dim or too harsh), heating (is it too hot or too cold), the layout of the room particularly where chairs are positioned around a table (can you move them to remove the barrier), where the windows are and doors onto a busy corridor, as well as the more obvious distraction caused by phones ringing or vibrating. It is extremely helpful to always try to have water available to offer, as well as discreetly located tissues when appropriate.

Eye-contact and body language

Eye-contact should never be intimidating; looking directly at the person we are listening to should not include holding eye-contact with them over extended periods of time. It requires awareness of the social and cultural identity of the person we are listening to, our wider facial expressions, gestures and body positioning. It is difficult to look directly into another person's eyes; we either look at one eye or the other. It can be useful to look at a triangular section between the eyebrows and the nose, which maintains an interested 'face to face' technique, while minimising the risk of intimidation and power imbalances.

For some, this approach can come naturally; however, for many of us, it is important to be aware of how we maintain eye-contact, if and how we gesture with our hands (this can be intimidating) and if our facial expression becomes static rather than engaged and encouraging. Roleplay with colleagues/peers definitely assists in developing and maintaining self-awareness.

Clarification and summarising

Checking out what you think the person has said to you assists both in achieving clarity of information and in demonstrating that you have been attentive and respectful. The basic *How? What? Who? When? Where?* format, when used in a positive and non-threatening way, assists in maintaining an open and non-leading approach to the gathering of information such as *'So, from what you have said, [action] supported you in the past. How do you think that can be achieved again?'* In general, we suggest that caution should be employed when asking *Why?* based questions as, in some situations, they may be received as blaming, leading and disempowering.

Professional curiosity

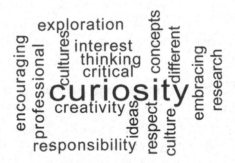

This concept is frequently cited, particularly in relation to safeguarding, both in children's serious case reviews and in safeguarding adults reviews. The following statement is included within *The Munro Review of Child Protection* undertaken during 2010 on behalf of HM Government, Department of Education.

Building strong relationships with children and families with compassion is crucial to reducing maltreatment, but trust needs to be placed with care, and 'respectful uncertainty' towards families, and interest and curiosity in their narratives, needs to be part of the practice mindset.

(Munro, 2010, p 18)

There was a lack of curiosity when faced with adults who used significant amounts of drugs and alcohol. Professionals did not establish their domestic circumstances or the implications for children living in the household and did not consider compromised parenting capacity.

(Stobart, 2017, p 8)

As previously suggested, in cases of alleged harm or neglect practitioners should consider if the person they are working with may be avoiding allowing access to their home environment; this may be due, for example, to factors of self-neglect, exploitation or coercive behaviours.

So, what is 'professional curiosity'?

As multidisciplinary teams and services do we have a commonality of language and understanding? A useful article was published in *The Nursing Times*, and as practitioners, we have found it to be a useful and concise set of questions, which encapsulate respectful, interested and empathetic professional curiosity:

It is essential for organisations to develop a culture of curiosity, which leads to ownership at every level – health professionals asking the right questions at each step of the way. [...]

These questions can help you to start practising curiosity:

> » *What happened?*
> » *When did it happen?*
> » *Where did it happen?*
> » *Why did it happen?*
> » *How might I...?*
> » *What if there was another possibility?*
> » *What else is available for me to choose... that I haven't chosen?*
> » *What skills, tools, relationships or other resources do I have or want for achieving my goals?*

(Oshikanlu, 2014, np)

In applying a respectful professionally curious approach to safeguarding, we should gather a clear picture of the person's life story and personal identity. This will involve questioning our own perspectives, opinions and personal as well as professional life experiences to ensure that we sensitively delve that little bit deeper to understand why the person may appear disengaged, passive, dismissive of the possibilities that things can change, or in denial that there is any sort of problem in the first place. The *SnapShots on...* included in this chapter give an initial insight and overview of the types of issues which can impact directly on how a person receives and accepts support through their safeguarding journey.

For those readers who are practitioners in social care, the *Professional Capabilities Framework* (PCF), originally developed by the Social Work Reform Board and now managed and delivered by the British Association of Social Workers (BASW, 2018), includes 'critical reflection and analysis' and 'professional leadership' as two of its nine elements. We have summarised both elements below based on different levels. This framework is also reproduced as Figure 2.4.

Critical Reflection (All Levels)

They use critical thinking augmented by creativity and **curiosity**.

Professional Leadership (Advanced and Strategic Levels)

Promote a culture of **professional curiosity** embracing research within your area of responsibility, encouraging the exploration of different cultures, concepts and ideas.

Figure 2.4 The BASW PCF

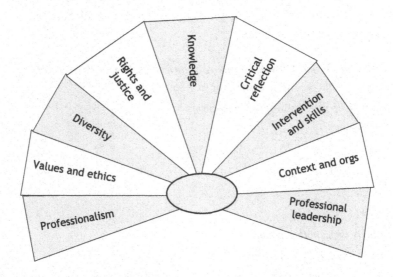

The BASW PCF (2018, p 6) includes the emphasis:

Our reflection enables us to challenge ourselves and others, and maintain our professional curiosity, creativity and self-awareness.

Professional, reflective practice supervision

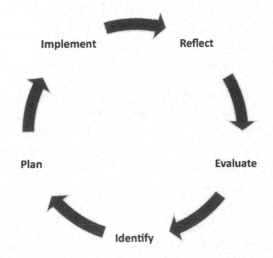

There are many and diverse approaches to what is often quite simply referred to as 'supervision'; it can include line management and employment-related issues such as when leave from work is planned to be taken, our time-management, as well as a time for the identification of learning and development needs. Here we are considering the role of critical and reflective practice supervision in the context of casework discussion and future planning.

As highlighted earlier, it is vitally important that we, as practitioners, take full responsibility for the critical review of our casework interventions and fully participate in what we refer to as 'reflective practice supervision' with our managers, as well as case discussions with peers and the wider multidisciplinary team/service.

The responsibility for ensuring that reflective practice supervision is real and meaningful does not, however, solely lie with the practitioner. As team and service managers, across all agencies, we also have a clear responsibility to ensure that support is provided to frontline practitioners which enables them to effectively and appropriately discharge their responsibilities. This level and type of support extends not only to the critical evaluation of each of the cases the practitioner is working on but also to ensuring that they are fully supported in positive risk-taking practices in line with organisational boundaries and expectations. Reflective practice supervision should be enabling and support creative, solution-focused thinking, with the arrangement of access to relevant subject matter experts such as lawyers, doctors, psychologists, the police, etc, when required.

As an aid to support reflective practice evaluation we have included, in Chapter 6, a simple recording tool, 'SnapShot on... MSP Practitioner "Reflective Practice" Resource' which we have found, as practitioners, to be of use not only for our own individual purposes but also as a support in preparing for reflective practice supervision. This resource can also be used in conjunction with the chronology template included in the 'SnapShot on... a chronology in safeguarding adults' below.

Learning from Life case scenarios

The adoption of active listening skills, respectful professional curiosity and a recognition of how early life experiences can impact upon adulthood enabled the development of the Learning from Life case scenarios.

Initial MSP approach: scenario one – JA

Limited information was available about JA's willingness to engage positively in response to the Safeguarding Concern raised. JA had, until approximately three years earlier, accepted low-level support, but had at that point disengaged and refused their involvement – he would turn the support worker away or not answer the door; the case was closed. It was very clear that all contacts must be pre-arranged with him by telephone, and that an unannounced visit to him at his home would be wholly inappropriate.

As described in Chapter 1, a combination of theory bases was adopted in planning case-work with JA; this included the design of a 'conversation framework' built upon elements of person-centred and relationship models. This initial conversation framework was constructed using a predominantly *What?* focused approach; examples include:

» What is important to you?

» What works well for you?

» What doesn't work so well?

» What could improve things for you?

Initial contact with JA showed that he was an extremely intelligent, articulate and well-educated person; however, it was learned that he was unable to engage in conversation which included any level of abstract thinking, such as '*What could improve things?*' In describing how this impacted upon the establishment of a positive and trusting relationship with JA, it took significant time investment in active listening, ongoing communication with him, particularly via the telephone, supported by the use of pictures and other graphic representations of the outcomes he wished to achieve. JA's own interpretation of what the MSP Principles meant to him personally are shown in Figure 2.5.

JA's life story board

During conversations with JA, the following story board was constructed:

Family unit and early life

Mother: Full-time carer of her children and home; she experienced episodes of severe depression which resulted in hospital admissions for treatment during JA's early/formative years.

Father: A senior accountant with a long-term dependency on alcohol; he died when JA was ten years old.

Sibling: Younger sister: no close or lasting relationship – they didn't engage together as children.

Social network: JA has no memories of mixing and playing with neighbours or classmates from school.

Adolescence and education

Home: Tensions due to JA's mother's mental ill-health. JA recollects that he found the role of elder sibling challenging.

School: High academic achiever at mainstream school; he obtained the A levels he needed to attend his chosen university.

University: Attended university at age 19 following his first admission to psychiatric inpatient care under Section 3 of the Mental Health Act (1983). JA experienced an acute episode of 'mania', with sleeplessness, pacing and compulsive handwashing; he received a diagnosis of schizophrenia. JA graduated from university with a first-class honour's degree.

Social network: JA continued with an isolated way of life, spending little time in social situations as his focus was solely upon his academic work. He describes that he had hypersensitivities to his environment at that time, which was later diagnosed as hyperacusis (intolerance of everyday sounds).

Adulthood

When JA graduated from university, he experienced his second episode of acute mental illness; 'mania' type behaviour re-emerged, with sleeplessness, pacing and compulsive handwashing. He was detained to a place of safety under Section 136 of the Mental Health Act (1983) and then transferred from Section 2 to Section 3 of the Act for medicines-based treatment to be given.

JA was discharged to 'hostel' style accommodation where he had his own room and received basic housing type support services – this arrangement was sustained for a period of over ten years. He was unable to secure any form of employment during this time and received welfare benefit payments.

JA experienced his third episode of acute mental illness; he displayed the same pattern of behaviours as he had previously, with the addition of intrusive thoughts and suicidal ideology – he attempted to jump from a bridge into the path of a train, but was restrained by police officers. A further admission into psychiatric hospital under Section 2, and medicines-based treatment under Section 3, followed. A diagnosis of 'autism' was made at that time (now recognised as '*6A02.0 Autism spectrum disorder without disorder of intellectual development and with mild or no impairment of functional language*', WHO, 2018).

On discharge, JA moved to a supported tenancy arrangement in closer proximity to his family home. Over a period of approximately six years, he became more socially isolated and refused the involvement of support services – he would turn them away or not answer the door. The home environment became increasingly cluttered and insanitary to the extent that complaints were made to the landlord. JA's mother was also increasingly concerned, and with the support of JA's sister privately arranged a short stay for JA at a care home while his home was cleaned and cleared – this short stay lasted nearly a year (the reasons for this are unknown). During this time his tenancy was maintained. However, he became more and more anxious to return home; he could have left of his own accord at any time.

When JA returned to his home address, the environment had been cleared and cleaned. On arrival he simply placed his belongings on the floor of the sitting room unpacked and returned to his 'hermit' like existence with the home environment again becoming insanitary and extremely cluttered – this continued for two years until the complaint made to the local Environmental Health department by his neighbour.

JA described how the neighbour had moved to live next door to him some years earlier and spent extended periods of time in the garden with music playing, mowing the lawn and using other pieces of noisy equipment. JA could not tolerate the noise, but the neighbour consistently refused to change how he used his garden. This disturbance obsessed JA, and he found it impossible to undertake his own everyday tasks.

Further relevant information

When JA is anxious, he will bang his head, slap himself, shout and swear to himself unpredictably. There are concerns that his teeth are badly decayed and causing him pain. JA doesn't use the central heating (because of the noise it makes) or electric lighting in the home. He has kept his curtains closed for several years because he is ashamed of the state of his home. He hasn't been able to use his bedroom, and although the toilet is functioning it is insanitary and extensively soiled.

Unless medicines or treatment are clearly described to him, using pictures or graphical aids, he will not accept them and will not follow recommended plans. There have also been suggestions that he may, at some point in the past, have been exploited by a person he thought was his friend; however, JA has added no details about this – he has simply stated that he doesn't want people coming to his home to take things from him.

Figure 2.5 Personalised MSP bubbles with JA

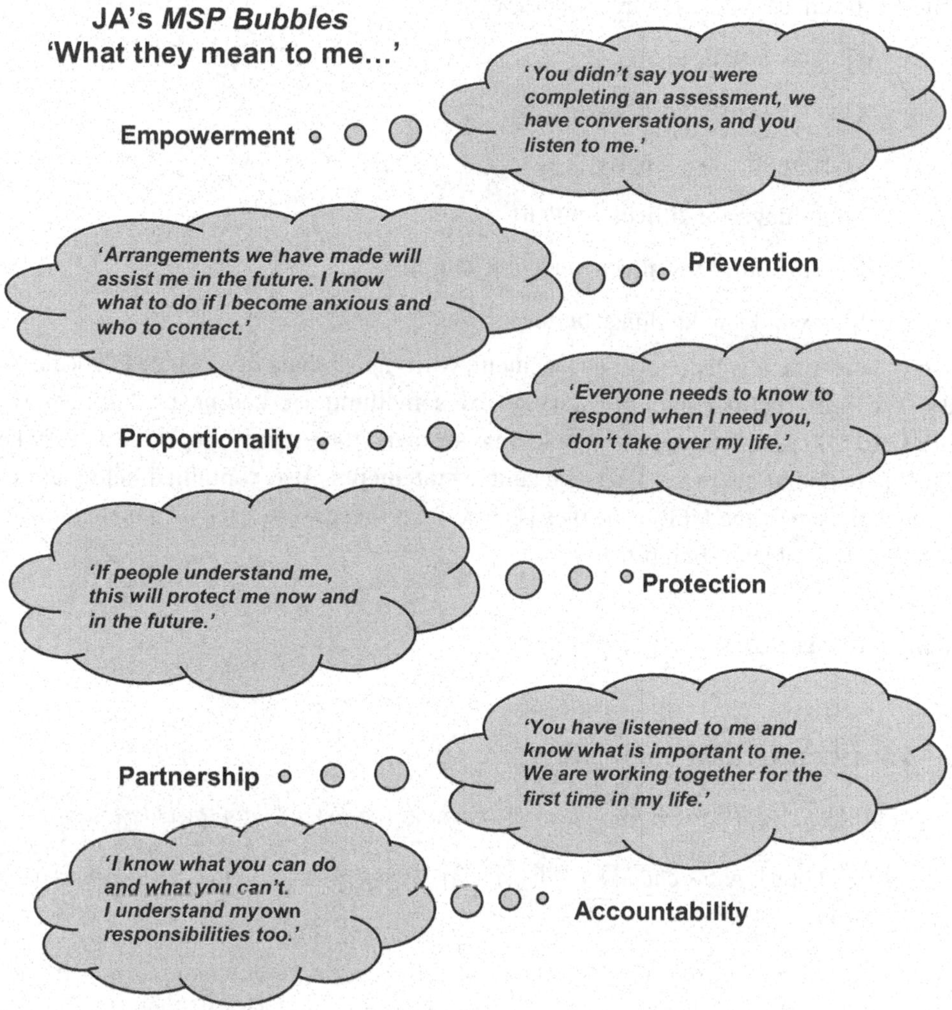

JA's *MSP Bubbles*
'What they mean to me...'

Empowerment

'*You didn't say you were completing an assessment, we have conversations, and you listen to me.*'

'*Arrangements we have made will assist me in the future. I know what to do if I become anxious and who to contact.*'

Prevention

'*Everyone needs to know to respond when I need you, don't take over my life.*'

Proportionality

'*If people understand me, this will protect me now and in the future.*'

Protection

'*You have listened to me and know what is important to me. We are working together for the first time in my life.*'

Partnership

'*I know what you can do and what you can't. I understand my own responsibilities too.*'

Accountability

Initial MSP approach: scenario two – CD

It is important to highlight that the local police had reviewed the details of the concern raised and confirmed that there was no evidence of criminal activity and the case was closed to them; however, in recognition of CD's known level of vulnerability, work was undertaken to establish an effective protection plan.

CD received a package of care and support co-ordinated by the local authority; she had also had support from an independent advocate when she moved to her current home.

As described above and in Chapter 1, a combination of theory bases was adopted in planning casework with CD, and a 'conversation framework' was developed as the basis for initial meetings. This was built upon elements of person-centred, relationship-based and solution-focused models.

CD was supported by an independent advocate during each meeting and, from early stages, it was possible to look at her solutions and desired outcomes; example questions included within this initial conversation framework were:

» What is working well?

» What isn't working so well?

» What could make it better?

» What things are difficult for you?

» Describe how they affect you living your life.

» What would make things better for you?

The initial exploratory process of engagement, with the support of a female advocate, enabled CD to construct her own life story board, something she had never done before. In response to CD's clear commitment to telling her own story, something she was very keen to do, it is included below as a set of example statements. Also contained below are CD's meanings of each of the MSP principles (Figure 2.6); these were used as a means to guide and explain the safeguarding process.

CD's life story board

> ## Family unit and early life
>
> *I am ... years old and I have two brothers and three sisters. I am the eldest.*
>
> *I haven't had a great childhood. All I've ever known is foster homes, care homes and hospitals.*
>
> *I wasn't brought up great. My dad was a very nasty man and he used to beat my mum for 15 years, and abused me mentally, physically and emotionally.*
>
> *There wasn't hugs or cuddles when I was younger, instead it was always getting belted all the time.*
>
> *My life changed when I was nine years old. I started to run away from home and that's when it started ... self-harming.*
>
> *This is the age when I started getting sexually abused by friends of the family and strangers who I thought I could trust.*
>
> *The only way I could block this out of my head is by self-harming. People started to wonder why this was happening. But I couldn't talk about what was happening to me. You see I thought this was the norm. I was put in to care at 11 years old because they thought I was beyond parental control.*

Adolescence

I was always running away. Taking overdoses and self-harming. But I couldn't tell anybody what was going on.

I had a son at 17 not long after I came out of care. He was a result of a rape. I brought him up until he was two years old then at 19, I had a nervous breakdown. I suppose my body and mind couldn't take it anymore.

They tried to bring me out of deep depression, but nothing really worked, then they gave me ECT [electroconvulsive therapy] and that worked.

Adulthood (from age 21)

After being three years in hospital I was getting ready to be discharged. I was told at 21 years old that [who] I thought was my dad wasn't really my dad. My mum was raped herself when she conceived me. It was hard when I found that out. I wasn't sure how I was feeling. I suppose I just felt numb inside. To this day I tell myself that I wish I wasn't told.

I feel like I'm a constant reminder to my mum about what happened to her. I still think about [it] every day and the more I think about it the more it hurts.

I've been in a lot of hospitals, some were OK some weren't. I've been in and out of hospitals for more than 20 years.

Things are looking up for me. I love my flat, it's the first proper home I've ever had.

I've had a boyfriend, he said that we would go on holiday, but it didn't happen. I was buying things for him, I wanted to. But he only came round when he wanted something, and I didn't like him bringing his friends round.

I started to cut myself again, and [support worker] saw it one day. She told me she was worried. I was worried when [support worker] saw my arm, but she told me it would be OK.

I don't know why [boyfriend] doesn't come round anymore really, but he said that he doesn't want to. I think it was because I told him that [support worker] was worried about me cutting again.

When the police came, I told them that I knew what I was doing, and no one was taking anything from me.

[Boyfriend] doesn't come here anymore – he won't come back. I miss him.

I need to focus on my trust with people, I know that not everybody in the world is BAD.

I do need a lot of help but I'm OK with [support worker].

Figure 2.6 Personalised MSP bubbles with CD

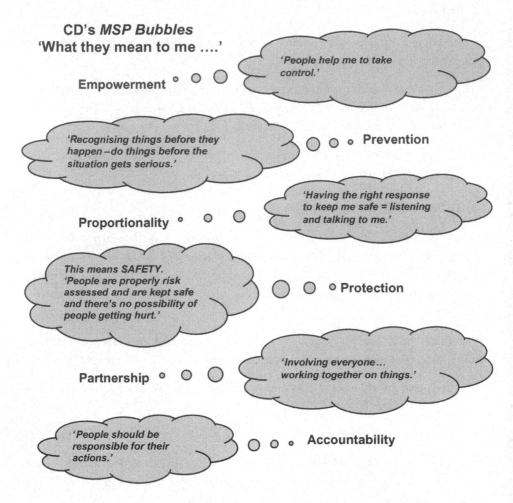

Further relevant information

CD has a diagnosis of paranoid schizophrenia and personality disorder. She is diabetic; this is tablet controlled. She is also morbidly obese, and experiences sleep apnoea.

Learning from Life case scenarios: summary

This chapter has been designed to give an overview and illustration of taking an MSP approach, with the bubble graphics included to add 'voices' to the translation of principles to everyday practice situations. The *SnapShots on...* included below address some of the issues of relevance to the Learning from Life case scenarios and are intended to prompt practitioners to research and explore the topics raised further as they choose.

The risks and strengths assessments completed, based upon the Learning from Life case scenarios, are detailed in Chapter 3, with associated safeguarding protection plans in Chapter 4.

Practice matters

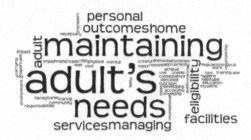

SnapShot on... **the Care Act (2014): eligible and non-eligible needs**

This *SnapShot* provides a precis of Chapter 10 of the *Care and Support Statutory Guidance* (Department of Health, 2018) to give practitioners a 'starter for ten' in the area of assessment, eligibility and planning.

Eligible needs

The Care Act (2014) says clearly that a person will be entitled to have their needs met when:

» the adult has 'eligible' needs (their eligible needs are those that are determined after the assessment);

» the adult is 'ordinarily resident' in the local area (which means their established home is there);

» any of five situations apply to them – these are set out in the Care and Support (Eligibility Criteria) Regulations 2015 (the 'eligibility regulations').

The five situations set out in the eligibility regulations are:

» the type of care and support they need is provided free of charge;

» the person cannot afford to pay the full cost of their care and support;

» the person asks the local authority to meet their needs;

» the person does not have mental capacity, and has no one else to arrange care for them;

» when the cap on care costs is introduced, their total care and support costs have exceeded the amount of the cap (confirmation in regulation continues to be awaited).

The eligibility regulations say an adult's needs meet the eligibility criteria if:

» the adult's needs arise from or are related to a physical or mental impairment or illness;

» as a result of the adult's needs the adult is unable to achieve two or more of the outcomes specified;

» as a consequence, there is, or is likely to be, a significant impact on the adult's well-being.

The specified outcomes are:

» managing and maintaining nutrition;

» maintaining personal hygiene;

» managing toilet needs;

» being appropriately clothed;

» being able to make use of the adult's home safely;

» maintaining a habitable home environment;

» developing and maintaining family or other personal relationships;

» accessing and engaging in work, training, education or volunteering;

» making use of necessary facilities or services in the local community including public transport, and recreational facilities or services; and

» carrying out any caring responsibilities the adult has for a child.

For the purposes of this regulation, an adult is to be regarded as being unable to achieve an outcome if the adult:

» is unable to achieve it without assistance;

» is able to achieve it without assistance but doing so causes the adult significant pain, distress or anxiety;

» is able to achieve it without assistance but doing so endangers or is likely to endanger the health or safety of the adult, or of others; or

» is able to achieve it without assistance but takes significantly longer than would normally be expected.

Where the level of an adult's needs fluctuates, in determining whether the adult's needs meet the eligibility criteria, the local authority must take into account the adult's circumstances over such period as it considers necessary to establish accurately the adult's level of need.

In considering the person's needs and how they may be met, the local authority must take into consideration any needs that are being met by a carer. The person may have assessed eligible needs which are being met by a carer at the time of the plan – in these cases the carer must be involved in the planning process. **Provided the carer remains willing and able to continue caring, the local authority is not required to meet those needs.** *However, the local authority should record the carer's willingness to provide care and the extent of this in the plan of the person and also the carer, so that the authority is able to respond to any changes in circumstances (for instance, a breakdown in the caring relationship) more effectively. Where the carer also has eligible needs, the local authority should consider combining the plans of the adult requiring care and the carer, if all parties agree, and establish if the carer requires an independent advocate.*

(Department of Health, 2018, para 10.40, emphasis added)

Non-eligible needs

Where a person has identified outcomes, which do not meet the threshold for the local authority to meet eligible needs (as described previously), these non-eligible needs should also be clearly recorded. Where all of the person's outcomes are confirmed as non-eligible needs – these should be clearly documented within the assessment and case records, with confirmation given to the person, or as applicable their representative:

in all cases the person must be given a written explanation of why their needs are not being met. The explanation provided to the person must be personal to and should be accessible for the person.

(Department of Health, 2018, para 10.29)

In some cases, non-eligible needs will form part of a broader Care and Support Plan which addresses eligible needs – in these cases, both sets of needs should be clearly documented within the Care and Support Plan and form part of all subsequent reviews. Some non-eligible needs may be met by the provision of information, advice or signposting to other agencies, community groups, etc.

This explanation must also include information and advice on how the person can reduce or delay their needs in future. This should be personal and specific advice based on the person's needs assessment and not a generalised reference to prevention services or signpost to a general web-site. For example, this should involve consideration of alternative ways in which a person could reduce or delay their care and support needs, including signposting to support within the local community.

(Department of Health, 2018, para 10.29)

Learning from Life case scenarios

Scenario one – JA

JA met the eligibility criteria in relation to the achievement of the following outcome areas:

» managing and maintaining nutrition;

» maintaining personal hygiene;

» being able to make use of the adult's home safely;

» maintaining a habitable home environment;

» developing and maintaining family or other personal relationships;

» accessing and engaging in work, training, education or volunteering;

» making use of necessary facilities or services in the local community including public transport, and recreational facilities or services.

Scenario two – CD

CD met the eligibility criteria in relation to the achievement of the following outcome areas:

» managing and maintaining nutrition;

» maintaining personal hygiene;

» being appropriately clothed;

» being able to make use of the adult's home safely;

» maintaining a habitable home environment;

» developing and maintaining family or other personal relationships;

» accessing and engaging in work, training, education or volunteering;

» making use of necessary facilities or services in the local community including public transport, and recreational facilities or services.

📸 *SnapShot on...* **advocacy in safeguarding and multicultural considerations**

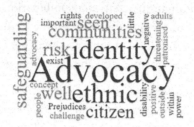

This *SnapShot* is designed to give practitioners an opportunity to extend their thinking in relation to advocacy to incorporate issues about cultural diversity.

Advocacy is an important concept for people from minority ethnic communities. Prejudices about disabled people exist within as well as outside minority ethnic communities and those with a disability often have little power, are patronised or seen as threatening. Through advocacy, citizen rights can be safeguarded, negative images challenged and positive identity developed.

(Mir et al, 2001, p 21)

Why is advocacy in safeguarding important within a multicultural context?

» Local authorities have a duty under Sections 67 and 68 of the Care Act (2014) to make available, and as required to provide, independent advocacy to adults who would experience **substantial difficulty** in being involved in care and support assessment and planning processes, a Safeguarding Enquiry or Safeguarding Adults Review (SAR) if:

  » an independent advocate was not provided then the person would have substantial difficulty in being fully involved in these processes;

  » there is no appropriate individual available to support and represent the person's wishes who is not paid or professionally engaged in providing care or treatment to the person or their carer.

» The Care Act (2014) defines four areas in which a **substantial difficulty** might be found. These are described within Chapter 6 of the *Care and Support Statutory Guidance* (Department of Health, 2018) as:

  » Understanding relevant information.

  » Retaining information.

  » Using or weighing up the information as part of the process of being involved.

  » Communicating their views, wishes and feelings.

» The concept of substantial difficulty must be judged for each person individually – considering each of the four factors noted above.

» People who are from Black and Minority Ethnic (BME) or Black, Asian and Minority Ethnic (BAME) communities may often face a combination of multiple factors of discrimination, such as a combination of race, disability, gender or sexual orientation. Advocacy can provide a vital link to services that are not always sensitive to their needs, thereby enabling marginalised and often disempowered individuals to speak up about their views and concerns.

» *'The concept of advocacy is itself problematic as it may not be widely or fully understood nor easily translatable for many black and minority ethnic communities'* (Fulton and Richardson, 2010, p 1). This concept is also raised by Baker and Wightman (2014) in their publication *Same Difference? Advocacy for People Who Have a Learning Disability from Black and Minority Ethnic Groups – a Guide to Good Practice* as a matter for close consideration when working with other underrepresented groups such as the Irish travelling community. This may be one of the reasons why service uptake can be low; service commissioners and providers, therefore, need to take this into consideration when planning any support to be provided in relation to any Safeguarding Enquiry, etc.

» Diversity of need among service users from Black and Minority Ethnic backgrounds is not always acknowledged or met. Awareness can be poor around basic issues such as the ethnicity of the local community, information needs, and the impact of cultural and spiritual values on decision-making, risk management and wider safeguarding issues.

» Where an Independent Mental Capacity Advocate (IMCA, Mental Capacity Act 2005) is already involved with an individual then, unless it is inappropriate, the same person/advocate should be used in relation to Care Act procedures.

Skills for advocates working with individuals from BME and BAME communities.

» Advocates should not be judgemental or make assumptions about the Safeguarding Concern/Enquiry based on their cultural background, language or gender but sensitively explore individual needs.

» Advocacy needs to challenge the double discrimination of racism and disability which can be experienced by adults at risk in BME and BAME communities.

» Advocacy should promote integration and facilitate access to culturally appropriate services.

» Advocacy should empower BME and BAME service users and their carers to identify their own needs in relation to Making Safeguarding Personal (MSP) and develop culturally appropriate ways to meet them.

» Advocates should take into consideration the cultural background, language and gender of the individuals they are supporting.

Terminology

The following definitions are taken from the Institute of Race Relations (IRR, nd):

Black – *The way that people of African descent describe themselves in countries such as South Africa, the US and parts of Europe. In the UK the term was also used (and can still be) in a political sense by other minority ethnic groups, especially Asians, who feel that their common experience of racism outweighs cultural differences.*

BME/BAME – *Black and Minority Ethnic or Black, Asian and Minority Ethnic is the terminology normally used in the UK to describe people of non-white descent.*

Culture – *The customs and mores of a particular nation, people or group.*

Learning from Life case scenarios

Scenario one – JA

An advocate with experience and skill in working with people with autism was arranged as JA had 'substantial difficulty' in fully participating and being involved. JA described that he would feel more supported if the gender of the advocate was female, and also if they were a similar age to himself.

Scenario two – CD

CD has previously been supported by a female advocate, with whom she had established a positive and supportive relationship. At the time advocacy support was required, this individual was available and appropriately trained to meet CD's need for support to be fully involved and to participate.

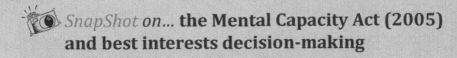

SnapShot on... the Mental Capacity Act (2005) and best interests decision-making

When to assess someone's mental capacity

Always document why a decision to assess the mental capacity of a person, aged 16 years or older, has been made, meeting each of the five principles contained within the Mental Capacity Act (2005).

1. *Presumption of capacity: A person must be assumed to have capacity unless it is established that he lacks capacity.*

2. *Advocacy and support: A person is not to be treated as unable to make a decision unless all practicable steps to help him to do so have been taken without success.*

3. *Human rights: A person is not to be treated as unable to make a decision merely because he makes an unwise decision.*

4. *Best interests: An act is done, or decision made, under this Act for or on behalf of a person who lacks capacity must be done, or made, in their best interests.*

5. *Less restrictive option: Before the act is done, or the decision is made, regard must be had to whether the purpose for which it is needed can be as effectively achieved in a way that is less restrictive of the person's rights and freedom of action.*

For example:

» A family member is concerned that their relative has become unable to make some more complex financial management decisions and they plan to register and use a Lasting Power of Attorney – Property and Financial Affairs.

» Concerns are raised because a person repeatedly makes unwise decisions that put them at significant risk of harm or exploitation or makes a particular unwise decision that is obviously irrational or out of character.

How to carry out a Mental Capacity Act (2005) assessment?

This follows what is called the 'two-stage test'.

Stage 1

The Mental Capacity Act (2005) requires confirmation that a person has an impairment of the mind or brain, or that there is some sort of disturbance affecting the way their mind or brain works (temporary or permanent); this does not require a formal medical diagnosis.

Impairment of the mind or brain, or disturbance affecting the way their mind or brain works, could include, for example, the side-effect of some forms of medicines which can include drowsiness, etc; a physical health condition which has caused a loss of consciousness, confusion, etc; an accident, trauma or brain injury; the effects of alcohol or drug use; or the symptoms of a mental health condition such as schizophrenia or dementia.

Stage 2

Does the impairment or disturbance of the mind or brain mean that the person is unable to make the decision in question at the time it needs to be made? In order for a person to be assessed as holding the mental capacity to make the specific decision at the time it needs to be made, the answer to each of the following four questions is 'yes':

1. Can the person **understand** information relevant to the decision to be made?

2. Can the person **retain** relevant information in their mind for as long as they need to make the decision?

3. Can the person **weigh up and balance** relevant factors for and against the decision?

4. Can the person **communicate** their decision (this includes all recognisable forms of communication, for example, the use of an interpreter, sign language, visual/pictorial aids)?

Evidence of how the person meets or fails to meet these four requirements must be clearly documented. If the answer to any one or all of the four elements is 'no', the person must be confirmed to lack the mental capacity to make the specified decision at the time it needs to be made.

Mental capacity should always be assessed for a particular decision at a particular time. In cases of people with 'fluctuating capacity', it may be appropriate and possible to discuss and agree with them the completion of a 'My Advance Support Plan – Choice and Control' (Britten and Whitby, 2018) of how they would like their needs to be met, and who they would like to be involved. This Advance Support Plan could then be of relevance, in relation to past wishes and preferences, if the need arose for a decision in their best interests to be made in the future.

How to make a best interests decision?

The person responsible for making a 'best interests decision' should be based on the individual circumstances of the case at the time a decision is needed, for example:

» Family members make decisions in many day-to-day situations. They may also act as the longer-term decision-maker regarding the care and treatment of the person who lacks capacity. The decision for medical treatment or social care will depend on the person who is responsible for that treatment and care. There are certain best interests decisions that cannot be made on behalf of a person who lacks the mental capacity to make the decision for themself. These include, for example, consenting to marriage or divorce; consenting to to having sexual relationships; consenting to a child being placed for adoption or the making of an adoption order; and a decision on voting at an election for any public office or at a referendum (not exhaustive/exclusive).

When making a best interests decision confirm:

1. What the decision to be made is: establish and confirm if an advanced decision, in relation to the specific issue under consideration, has already been made.

2. Why does the decision have to be made at this time: consider and confirm if the decision can be put off until the person regains capacity.

3. How the person is being involved: assumptions about a person's best interests should not be made on the basis of their age, appearance, behaviour, and/or all relevant protected characteristics.

4. Who is involved in identifying what the best interests of the person are: consider and confirm all relevant circumstances and information (past preferences, wishes and beliefs, etc).

5. Evidence how all options have been evaluated (factors for and against) and clearly document the basis for the decision made is the less restrictive option.

Proforma best interests decision recording template

Option one	
Add details of the option HERE	
Positive aspects *(for)*	**Negative aspects** *(against)*
Option two	
Add details of the option HERE	
Positive aspects *(for)*	**Negative aspects** *(against)*
Option three	
Add details of the option HERE	
Positive aspects *(for)*	**Negative aspects** *(against)*

Less restrictive option
Add details of the decision HERE

Learning from Life case scenarios

Scenario one – JA

Concerns were raised that JA may lack the mental capacity to make the decision to have his home environment cleaned and made safe. A Mental Capacity Act (2005) assessment was completed. This assessment established that with the support of an advocate and with information provided in both linear and pictorial formats he was able to demonstrate that he could understand, retain, weigh in the balance and communicate his decision.

Scenario two – CD

There were no concerns about CD's mental capacity; the requirement for a presumption of capacity was met (a person must be assumed to have capacity unless it is established that they lack capacity).

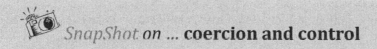 *SnapShot* on ... **coercion and control**

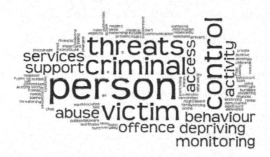

This *SnapShot* is designed to give practitioners a starting point from which to explore and further expand their knowledge and understanding of this complex and highly serious criminal offence under the Serious Crime Act (2015) in England and Wales. It also suggests further reading materials which place the concept of coercive controlling behaviour, and its impact, as a matter of global importance which crosses geographic, social and cultural boundaries. An extremely accessible and valuable resource is a book published in 2018 by two brothers, Luke and Ryan Hart, who directly experienced coercive behaviour within their own home and family, which very sadly resulted in the deaths of their mother and sister at the hands of their father (who also killed himself) – *Operation Lighthouse: Reflections on our Family's Devastating Story of Coercive Control and Domestic Homicide.*

The criminal offence

The Serious Crime Act (2015) created a criminal offence of controlling or coercive behaviour in ongoing intimate or familial relationships where, at the time the behaviour occurs, the perpetrator and victim are personally connected – this offence is contained within Section 76 of that Act (HM Government, 2015b). The *Statutory Guidance Framework* (Home Office, 2015a) states that behaviour must have occurred on at least two occasions and have had:

» a serious effect *or*

» substantial adverse effect on the victims' day to day activities *and*

» the alleged perpetrator must have known that their behaviour would have a serious effect on the victim *or*

» they ought to have known it would have that effect.

It is important to note that this criminal offence specifically relates to behaviour by the perpetrator that happens 'repeatedly or continuously' (Home Office, 2015a, Section 1); a successful prosecution can result in a maximum custodial sentence of five years, a fine or both.

The cross-government definition of domestic violence and abuse (this is not a legal definition and includes so-called 'honour'-based violence, female genital mutilation (FGM) and forced marriage, and is clear that victims are not confined to one gender or ethnic group) outlines controlling or coercive behaviour as follows.

» **Controlling behaviour** *is a range of acts designed to make a person subordinate and/or dependent by isolating them from sources of support, exploiting their resources and capacities for personal gain, depriving them of the means needed for independence, resistance and escape and regulating their everyday behaviour.*

» **Coercive behaviour** *is a continuing act or a pattern of acts of assault, threats, humiliation and intimidation or other abuse that is used to harm, punish, or frighten their victim.*

The types of behaviours associated with coercion or control may or may not constitute a criminal offence in their own right. It is important to remember that the presence of controlling or coercive behaviours does not mean that no other offence has been committed or cannot be charged. However, the perpetrator may limit space for action and exhibit a story of ownership and entitlement over the victim. Such behaviours might include:

» *isolating a person from their friends and family;*

» *depriving them of their basic needs;*

» *monitoring their time;*

» *monitoring a person via online communication tools or using spyware;*

» *taking control over aspects of their everyday life, such as where they can go, who they can see, what to wear and when they can sleep;*

» *depriving them of access to support services, such as specialist support or medical services;*

» *repeatedly putting them down such as telling them they are worthless;*

» *enforcing rules and activity which humiliate, degrade or dehumanise the victim;*

» *forcing the victim to take part in criminal activity such as shoplifting, neglect or abuse of children to encourage self-blame and prevent disclosure to authorities;*

» *financial abuse including control of finances, such as only allowing a person a punitive allowance;*

» *threats to hurt or kill;*

» *threats to a child;*

» *threats to reveal or publish private information (eg threatening to 'out' someone).*

» *assault;*

» *criminal damage (such as destruction of household goods);*

» *rape;*

» *preventing a person from having access to transport or from working.*

This is not an exhaustive list.

(Home Office, 2015a, Section 2)

Research and current developments

The vast majority of research (worldwide) into domestic violence in intimate or familial relationships has emphasised gender-focused aspects upon men as the perpetrator of violence.

Women as well as men physically assault their partners. But coercive control is 'gendered' because it is used to secure male privilege and its regime of domination/subordination is constructed around the enforcement of gender stereotypes. 'Domination' here refers to both the power/privilege exerted through coercive control in individual relationships and to the political power created when men as a group use their oppressive tactics to reinforce persistent sexual inequalities in the larger society.

(Stark, 2012, np)

Research and publications date back to the mid-twentieth century and include works by the late Susan Schechter (Coalition Against Domestic Violence, Denver, Colorado) from the 1980s and Evan Stark, Professor Emeritus, Rutgers University, New Jersey. Walklate et al (2017) record that '*Evan Stark's (2007, 2009) work is critical to recent understandings of coercive control and moves to criminalise it'*, while recognising that the definition used as part of the Serious Crime Act (2015) is neutral in terms of gender and ethnicity.

the form of subjugation that drives most abused women to seek outside assistance is not encompassed by the violence model and that, therefore, interventions predicated on this model are ineffective in protecting women and children from this type of abuse. These women have been subjected to a pattern of domination that includes tactics to isolate, degrade, exploit and control them as well as to frighten them or hurt them physically. This pattern, which may include but is not limited to physical violence, has been variously termed psychological or emotional abuse, patriarchal or intimate terrorism (Tolman, 1992; Johnson, 2008), and coercive control (Stark, 2007), the term I prefer.

(Stark, 2012, p 120)

This 2012 work of Stark's incorporates research conducted in Britain with a group of 500 women who sought help from Refuge UK, published in 2006 (Rees et al, 2006). Interestingly, the overwhelming majority of women who took part in this survey reported intimidating, humiliating and degrading behaviours from their partner when compared with reports of physically violent behaviours; these are summarised below:

Emotionally focused behaviours:

  » 96 per cent reported that their partners called them names.

  » 94 per cent reported that their partners swore at them.

  » 95 per cent reported that their partners brought up things from their past to hurt them.

  » 97 per cent reported that their partners *'said something to spite me'*.

  » 93 per cent reported that their partners *'ordered me around'*.

Violent behaviours:

  » 70 per cent had been choked or strangled at least once.

  » 60 per cent had been beaten in their sleep.

  » 24 per cent had been cut or stabbed at least once.

  » Almost 60 per cent had been forced to have sex against their will.

  » 26.5 per cent had been 'beaten unconscious'.

  » 10 per cent had been 'tied up'.

  » 38 per cent of the women reported suffering 'permanent damage'.

In the UK, on 22 October 2018, the House of Commons, Home Affairs Committee published the *Domestic Abuse: Ninth Report of Session 2017–2019*. The Home Affairs Committee is appointed by the House of Commons to examine the expenditure, administration and policy of the Home Office and its associated public bodies. This report is the outcome of a short inquiry into the government's proposed draft Domestic Abuse Bill; it included written consultation submissions as well as 'face to face' meetings. The finalised groundbreaking Domestic Abuse Bill, updated following consultation submissions, had its first reading in the House of Commons on 3 March 2020. A selection of issues discussed is included below.

A statutory definition of domestic abuse

Paragraph 10

The Government wants to ensure that all domestic abuse is properly understood, considered unacceptable and actively challenged across statutory agencies and in public attitudes. One of the measures which it proposes is to introduce a new statutory definition of domestic abuse which covers all victims and all types of domestic abuse. (8) The proposed definition includes wider family members as well as couples, and it aims to include the many different types of behaviour which can be exhibited as part of domestic abuse. The proposed definition includes the following text:

> *Any incident or pattern of incidents of controlling, coercive, threatening behaviour, violence or abuse between those aged 16 or over who are, or have been, intimate partners or family members regardless of gender or sexual orientation. The abuse can encompass but is not limited to psychological; physical; sexual; economic; emotional.*

Gendered nature of domestic abuse

Paragraph 11

In its consultation paper, the Government referred to the close links between its domestic abuse and its Violence Against Women and Girls (VAWG) strategies and noted that on a global level, domestic abuse is one of the most endemic forms of violence against women. It said that it aimed to use the draft bill on domestic abuse to demonstrate the Government's commitment to ratifying the Istanbul Convention by extending extraterritorial jurisdiction over VAWG related offences. It also acknowledged the gendered nature of domestic abuse:

> *We know that domestic abuse is disproportionately gendered and have framed our consultation to recognise this. Equally, this is why our approach to tackling domestic abuse remains within the context of a wider Violence Against Women and Girls Strategy. The majority of domestic abuse victims are women, with men far more likely to be perpetrators.*

Women's Aid and Amnesty International UK were part of this inquiry and submitted a range of evidence for consideration. We have included here a couple of excerpts from their evidence which we feel will be of use to practitioners, and add to an understanding of coercive control in the context of domestic abuse (emphasis has been added by the authors):

Paragraph 14

Witnesses also argued that the gendered nature of domestic abuse should be recognised in the statutory definition so as to provide the best possible protection to survivors and to comply with

VAWG legislation and policies. Councillor Simon Blackburn, representing the Local Government Association, described domestic abuse as 'a heavily gendered crime'. Women's Aid explained that as well as women being more likely than men to be victims of domestic abuse, the nature and impact of men's abuse towards women was qualitatively different. **Women were more likely to experience fear, be subject to coercive control, experience repeat victimisation** *and were far more likely to be killed. It explained that gender-neutral services failed to deliver the gender-specific support required by victims of abuse. Amnesty International UK provided the following statistics:*

> *According to data collected in 2016 and 2017 by the Office of National Statistics women are around twice as likely as men to experience domestic violence, and men are far more likely to be perpetrators. Most domestic homicide victims are women, killed by men. On average, two women are killed each week by their current or former partner in England and Wales, a figure that has changed relatively little in recent years. Between March 2014 and 2016, 242 women were killed by a male partner/ex-partner; 32 men were killed by their male partner/ex-partner, and 40 by their female partner/ex-partner.*

Practitioner toolkit

We have found the following two graphic representations (Figure 2.7 and Figure 2.8) created by the Domestic Abuse Intervention Programs (DAIP) in Duluth, Minnesota, USA, when used in conjunction, to be of use to us in practice. *The Duluth Model*, as it came to be known, was first developed in the 1980s by a group of community-based agencies who work to end violence against women. Their work has extended across the globe, and advocates the following values as their core mission.

1. *We listen to battered women: Our work involves active engagement with women who have experienced violence so that our efforts are guided by their realities and concerns.*

2. *We educate to promote liberation: An educational process of dialogue and critical thinking is key to our efforts to assist women in understanding and confronting the violence directed against them, and to our efforts to challenge and support men who commit to ending battering.*

3. *We advocate for institutional and social change: We examine the practices and policies of social and governmental agencies that intervene in the lives of battered women and address systemic problems by engaging with institutional practitioners and leaders in the development of creative and effective solutions.*

4. *We struggle against all forms of oppression. Women are not defined by a single identity, but live in the intersection of their race, gender, class, ethnicity, nationality, disability, age, religion and sexual orientation. Our work must also challenge all systems of oppression that create a climate of supremacy and intolerance that facilitates violence and exploitation in women's lives.*

5. *We promote non-violence and peace: Every step we take, every interaction we have with others, is an opportunity to advance non-violence, continually working toward and building a culture and a future of peace.*

The first graphic (Figure 2.7) shows the interplay and facets of power and control; the second (Figure 2.8) details further consideration of organisational/institutional discrimination which can occur through a lack of recognition of culture, ethnicity and personal identity. These tools can act as a useful resource for practitioners to add to their 'practice toolkit' when balanced with further recognition of the impacts individual and combined protected characteristics (Equality Act 2010) can have on a person's experiences of life when not respected.

Figure 2.7 Facets of power and control DAIP (1980)

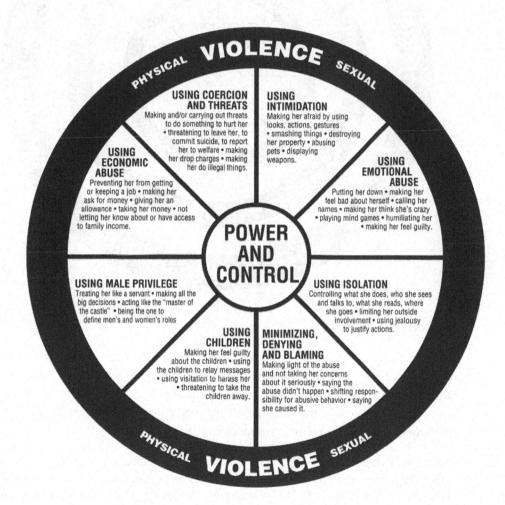

Figure 2.8 Considerations in organisational/institutional discrimination DAIP (1980)

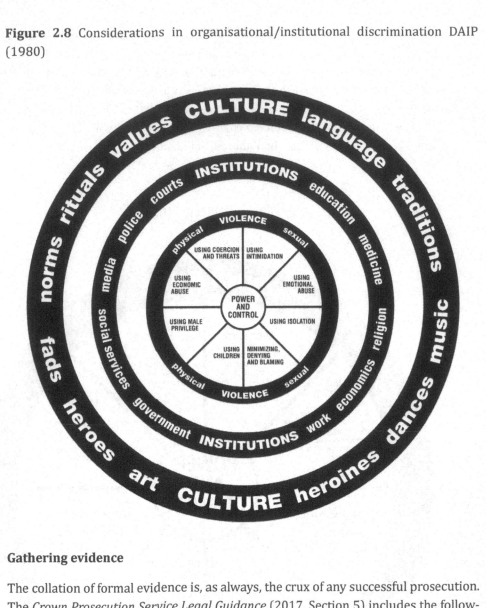

Gathering evidence

The collation of formal evidence is, as always, the crux of any successful prosecution. The *Crown Prosecution Service Legal Guidance* (2017, Section 5) includes the following guidance to support the collection of relevant evidence upon which a case of coercive control can be built. It also signposts to further information contained within the *Statutory Guidance Framework* (Home Office, 2015a):

Efforts aimed at gathering evidence to build a robust prosecution case should focus on the wider pattern of behaviour and on the cumulative impact on a person. It should also be noted that a victim may not know the full extent of a perpetrator's conduct therefore all potential lines of enquiry should be explored.

» *Copies of emails*

» *Phone records*

» *Text messages*

» *Evidence of abuse over the internet, digital technology and social media platforms*

» *Photographs of injuries such as defensive injuries to forearms, latent upper arm grabs, scalp bruising, clumps of hair missing*

» *999 tapes or transcripts*

» *CCTV*

» *Body-worn video footage*

» *Lifestyle and household including at scene photographic evidence*

» *Records of interaction with services such as support services, (even if parts of those records relate to events which occurred before the new offence came into force, their contents may still, in certain circumstances, be relied on in evidence)*

» *Medical records*

» *Witness testimony, for example, the family and friends of the victim may be able to give evidence about the effect and impact of isolation of the victim from them*

» *Local enquiries: neighbours, regular deliveries, postal, window cleaner etc*

» *Bank records to show financial control*

» *Previous threats made to children or other family members*

» *Diary kept by the victim*

» *Victims account of what happened to the police*

» *Evidence of isolation such as lack of contact between family and friends, victim withdrawing from activities such as clubs, perpetrator accompanying victim to medical appointments*

» *GPS tracking devices installed on mobile phones, tablets, vehicles etc.*

» *Where the perpetrator has a carer responsibility, the care plan might be useful as it details what funds should be used for*

Even where there is a decision to take no further action, prosecutors should ask police officers to advise the victim to take steps to gather records to support any future investigation. This might include:

» *A diary of events (ideally in a bound book or timed by keeping an electronic record) noting that there are potential risks to the victim if the perpetrator were to discover this;*

» *Safely noting details of witnesses who may have observed or heard these events;*

» *Storing messages or taping calls made by the defendant;*

» *Safely speaking to neighbours, colleagues, family, friends or specialist support services*

However, note that it might be particularly difficult for some disabled people in receipt of informal or employed care support to gather evidence.

The police should advise the victim how to keep information about incidents and themselves safe. In addition, they should also signpost the victim to specialist domestic abuse services such as the 24 Hour National Domestic Violence Helpline (run in partnership by Women's Aid and Refuge on 0808 2000247).

📷 *SnapShot on...* **exploitation, 'county lines' and 'cuckooing'**

The Modern Slavery Act (2015) enhanced and formalised actions to be taken in order that the criminal justice system effectively prosecutes criminals and protects victims of slavery and/or trafficking.

This includes slavery, servitude and forced or compulsory labour; sexual exploitation; removal of organs; securing services etc by force, threats or deception; **and securing services etc** *from children and* **vulnerable persons.**

(Home Office, 2015b, p 6)

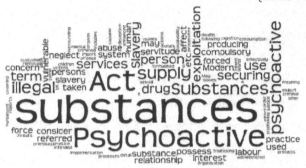

Psychoactive substances

More and more reports are covering the issues surrounding the availability and use of these illegal psychoactive substances following the implementation of the Psychoactive Substances Act (2016) which came into force from 26 May 2016 in the UK. This Act of Parliament:

makes it an offence to produce, supply, offer to supply, possess with intent to supply, possess on custodial premises, import or export psychoactive substances; that is, any substance intended for human consumption that is capable of producing a psychoactive effect.

(Home Office, 2018, np)

The World Health Organization (WHO, 2019) details the meaning of psychoactive substances as follows:

Psychoactive substances are substances that, when taken in or administered into one's system, affect mental processes, eg cognition or affect. This term and its equivalent, psychotropic drug are the most neutral and descriptive term for the whole class of substances, licit and illicit, of interest to drug policy. 'Psychoactive' does not necessarily imply dependence-producing, and in common parlance, the term is often left unstated, as in 'drug use' or 'substance abuse'.

In practice, involvement and contact, always consider whether the Modern Slavery Act (2015) and/or the Psychoactive Substances Act (2016) may apply – consider if the person you are working with may be being exploited by the securing of services from them. This could include the person acting as a courier of illegal substances – commonly referred to as 'county lines'; their home being used for the purposes of storing and/or the supplying of illegal substances – referred to as 'cuckooing'; or the person being used as a 'guinea pig' to test out the effects of new chemically created psychoactive substances.

Of particular interest, and matter of concern to us, is the relationship between abuse, neglect, self-neglect, exploitation of 'vulnerable persons' and the supply/use of illegal drugs and substances (also known as new psychoactive substances, NPS). There is little, if any, formal research into this relationship; however, based upon our practice experience, there exists both a clear cause for concern and need for greater understanding of this issue.

Under the Care Act (2014), local authorities have functions to make sure that people who live in their areas:

» receive services that prevent their care needs from becoming more serious or delay the impact of their needs;

» can get the information and advice they need to make good decisions about care and support;

» have a range of provision of high-quality, appropriate services to choose from.

This *SnapShot* poses the hypothesis that there is a causational relationship between the following factors (Figure 2.9) which compounds and exacerbates the risk of serious harm occurring; we actively encourage formal research to be initiated.

Figure 2.9 Factorial relationships of risk

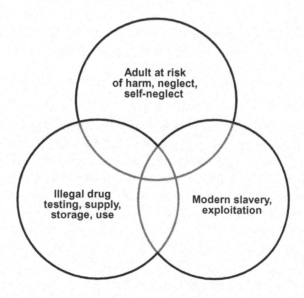

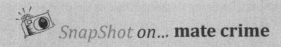

SnapShot on... **mate crime**

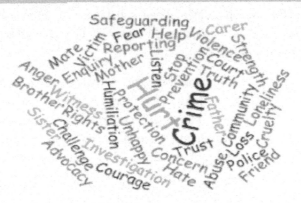

There is no statutory definition of 'mate crime' in UK law; the term is generally understood to refer to the befriending of people who are perceived by the perpetrator/source of harm to be vulnerable for the purposes of exploiting and/or abusing them; this may be associated with criminal offences of disability hate crime (Criminal Justice Act 2003, Section 146). This can be strongly associated, but not exclusively, with people with learning difficulties, learning disabilities or mental health conditions. The graphic above shows some of the words associated with mate crime.

Mate crime can resonate with cases of domestic abuse but involves additional complex issues. The perpetrator/source of harm can be perceived by the victim to be a trusted friend, carer or family member; they will use this relationship as a means for exploitation. Safeguarding Adults Reviews (previously called Serious Case Reviews) provide a useful description and important information for all practitioners; useful resources are included within the *Taking It Further* section at the end of this chapter.

The following text is an excerpt from the Hampshire Safeguarding Adults Board (nd) 'Safeguarding Adults Reviews' library; it demonstrates the relevance of the Human Rights Act (1998) in practice:

Hounslow Ruling

A High Court ruling in which the local authority was ordered to pay damages to a vulnerable family who had been abused by a gang of youths. This judgment concerns a claim for damages brought by a married couple with learning disabilities against Hounslow for negligence and breach of duty of care on the part of the local authority. They claimed the local authority failed to move them from their home using its emergency transfer procedure which could have prevented them from being subject to a horrific incident in their own home. They also were claiming damages under the Human Rights Act, 1998 (Sections 6 and 7) from the local authority because it failed to protect them from inhuman and degrading treatment, and to maintain the integrity of their private and family life, thus breaching Articles 3 and 8 respectively of the European Convention on Human Rights.

A person experiencing mate crime can be unaware of the perpetrator's motives and feel unable to challenge or exert control to change their situation of hurt and abuse.

Some features and signs of 'mate crime'

It can be difficult to recognise and intervene in cases of mate crime as it is often a pattern of repeat or worsening abuse which has occurred before any concerns are highlighted. The victim may experience:

» fear of reporting – the person may not recognise that what is happening is wrong, and they may be afraid of the consequences of disclosing;

» social isolation from their usual social contacts or sudden changes in their social network;

» lack of support – people who are targeted may often be those who do not meet threshold criteria for a high level of support from statutory agencies;

» coercion, intimidation or threats from their abuser as a means of control;

» withdrawal or removal from their usual social routines;

» unexplained physical injuries;

» lack of access to their money – bills may not be paid;

» changes in mood and physical presentation – more aggressive or more withdrawn, weight loss, deterioration in personal appearance.

The perpetrator/source of harm may expose their victim to one or more of the following forms of abuse:

» financial;

» emotional;

» physical;

» criminal exploitation;

» sexual.

In many situations, mate crime may be an example of disability hate crime and as such should be reported to the police, with a safeguarding adults concern submitted to the local safeguarding adults team.

Learning from Life case scenarios

Scenario one – JA

Mate crime was considered in relation to JA as a part of the development of his protection planning – he was clear that he felt vulnerable to people coming to his home and taking things from him; he did not provide details of actual events he said had occurred.

Scenario two – CD

The potential for CD to be exploited, and her personal vulnerability, were fundamental components in the development of her personal protection plan; this included enabling supported access to local awareness-raising and resilience training.

 SnapShot on... **a chronology in safeguarding adults**

The use of a chronology is frequently advocated as an effective approach to person-centred practice in all aspects of health and social care. This form of approach is of particular use in safeguarding adults enquiries as well as in cases when a practitioner is requested to submit evidence to a coroner (see Chapter 5, '*SnapShot on...* the coroner and reports under Regulation 28'), or in cases where a dispute between practitioners or their agencies arises (see Chapter 5, '*SnapShot on ...* dispute resolution').

If a practitioner has begun a chronology from the point at which they became involved in a case it can assist greatly in understanding the life story of the adult and their journey through life which arrives at their involvement with care and support services and their current situation.

The adoption of a 'professionally curious' approach to social care interventions can be supported by the review and analysis of a chronological record to identify elements of key importance and relevance to the adult.

The example chronology template contained below (Table 2.1) gives a clear and concise framework for use by all practitioners. The entries should start from the earliest known relevant information about the adult; in some cases, this will be from when they were a child and others at a point in their adult life. It is important to be concise in all recordings, using the 'Comment/significance' column to highlight events that appear to be pivotal; this will aid future reference and analysis. This is of particular relevance in cases of self-neglect where adults may have experienced trauma in their early years that has impacted upon their experiences and responses in adulthood.

Table 2.1 Example chronology template

Name of adult:
Date of birth:
Chronology period:
Agency name and address:
Name of author:
Designation of author:
Prepared for:

Date	Source of evidence	Name and designation of professional	Event/involvement/activity	Actions taken and decisions made	Comment/ significance
//**** (start with the earliest date)	Eg, case file record, letter, report	Ann Bloggs, social worker	Clear and concise details of the activity or involvement; eg, referral received from X about Y. When recording the time of an event(s) use the 24-hour clock format; ie, 13.00 hrs not 1 pm. Include facts, **not** assumptions or personal opinions. If you have been given information, confirm the source. Be clear if you have directly witnessed an event(s). Avoid jargon, acronyms or abbreviations – unless the meaning is clearly described. When referring to others include their name and role/designation.	**Who, what, where, when, why, how?** Clear and concise details of decisions reached and why. Actions taken and those planned. When referring to others include their name and role/designation.	Confirm professional judgement – highlighting as applicable the significance of the event.

NB: **Always include page numbers – Page 1 of 2, etc.**

As social workers and operational managers we have frequently been required to create chronologies for our own casework and with colleagues; in this we have found that the sooner you adopt this form of practice the less time you will have to spend in the future piecing information together. However, it is fully recognised that a proportionate approach, based upon professional judgement, should always be adopted.

Conclusion: overarching considerations in MSP

» Recognition of the fundamental needs which may be relevant to a person with an invisible or not clearly understood disability (eg, Asperger's Syndrome, hearing impairment, rare neurological condition).

» The engagement of active listening skills to understand and speak/communicate with the person based upon their perception of what the problem is; not imposing your own perceptions.

» The experience the adult may have had of disempowerment, discrimination and oppression as part of their life story; this could have been compounded upon further by the approach taken to address the Safeguarding Concern raised. It is vital that this is not perpetuated by the enquiry process and the perceived actions of the practitioner.

» Building a trust relationship by being an engaged, empathetic, interested and reliable practitioner.

» The provision of appropriate and culturally sensitive advocacy support with those people who would have 'substantial difficulty' in engaging and being involved in any safeguarding process (Department of Health, 2018, para 7.5).

» The principles and statutory requirements of the Mental Capacity Act (2005) – including:

  » critical consideration of fluctuations in a person's mental capacity to make decisions;

  » the fundamental right of a person to make what others may consider to be unwise decisions/choices.

» Issues of coercion or influence (eg, pressure from family members, friends/associates, carers, etc).

» Rights and risks: this could include the misinterpretation of a person's needs and capacity to make decisions simply because they are articulate; are there issues of fluctuations in mental capacity which could be addressed through advance planning with the person (eg, self-neglect which presents a known risk of serious harm or death may require a multi-agency risk management meeting to be convened, with the person attending wherever possible, rather than an assumption that they are simply making unwise choices)?

» Careful consideration and explanation of what realistically can be achieved; mitigate the risk of unrealistic expectations – be open, honest and fact-focused within applicable parameters (eg, it is not possible for the practitioner to pursue criminal proceedings where the police have made it clear that in law they will not).

» If the issue(s) that have arisen in work with a person have wider relevance and need to be escalated, ensure that this is actioned through your practice supervision – this could relate, for example, to learning and development initiatives, support service provision, the need for the availability of more diverse translator services, accessibility of information resources, communication systems, etc.

Taking it further

References

Baker, N and Wightman, C (2014) *Same Difference? Advocacy for People Who Have a Learning Disability from Black and Minority Ethnic Groups – a Guide to Good Practice.* Coventry: British Institute of Learning Disabilities (BILD). [online] Available at: www.bild.org.uk/EasySiteWeb/GatewayLink.aspx?alId=4209 (accessed 21 September 2020).

British Association of Social Workers (BASW) (2018) *Professional Capabilities Framework (PCF).* Birmingham: BASW. [online] Available at: www.basw.co.uk/system/files/resources/PCF%20Final%20Documents%20Overview%20 11%20June%202018.pdf (accessed 21 September 2020).

Britten, S and Whitby, K (2018) *Self-neglect: A Practical Approach to Risks and Strengths Assessment.* St Albans: Critical Publishing.

Crown Prosecution Service (reviewed 2017) *Controlling or Coercive Behaviour in an Intimate or Family Relationship Legal Guidance, Domestic Abuse.* London: Code for Crown Prosecutors, Director of Public Prosecutions. [online] Available at: www.cps.gov.uk/legal-guidance/controlling-or-coercive-behaviour-intimate-or-family-relationship (accessed 21 September 2020).

Department for Constitutional Affairs (2007) *The Mental Capacity Act (2005) Code of Practice.* Norwich: The Stationery Office (TSO). [online] Available at: www.gov.uk/government/publications/mental-capacity-act-code-of-practice (accessed 21 September 2020).

Department of Health (2018) *Care and Support Statutory Guidance.* [online] Available at: www.gov.uk/government/ publications/care-act-statutory-guidance/care-and-support-statutory-guidance (accessed 21 September 2020).

Domestic Abuse Intervention Programs (DAIP) (1980) *The Duluth Model.* Duluth, MN: DAIP. [online] Available at: www.theduluthmodel.org/wheels/ (accessed 21 September 2020).

Fulton, R and Richardson, K (2010) *Towards Race Equality in Advocacy Services: People with Learning Disabilities from BME Communities.* Better Health Briefing 15. London: Race Equality Foundation.

Hampshire Safeguarding Adults Board (nd) *Learning from Experience Database: Hounslow Ruling.* [online] Available at: www.hampshiresab.org.uk/learning-from-experience-database/serious-case-reviews/location/ hounslow/ (accessed 21 September 2020).

Hart, L and Hart, R (2018) *Operation Lighthouse: Reflections on our Family's Devastating Story of Coercive Control and Domestic Homicide.* London: Orion Publishing Group.

HM Government (1983) *Mental Health Act 1983.* Norwich: The Stationery Office. [online] Available at: www.legislation.gov.uk/ukpga/1983/20/pdfs/ukpga_19830020_en.pdf (accessed 21 September 2020).

HM Government (1998) *Human Rights Act 1998.* Norwich: The Stationery Office. [online] Available at: www.legislation.gov.uk/ukpga/1998/42/pdfs/ukpga_19980042_en.pdf (accessed 21 September 2020).

HM Government (2003) *Criminal Justice Act 2003.* Norwich: The Stationery Office. [online] Available at: www.legislation.gov.uk/ukpga/2003/44/pdfs/ukpga_20030044_en.pdf (accessed 21 September 2020).

HM Government (2010) *Equality Act 2010*. Norwich: The Stationery Office. [online] Available at: www.legislation. gov.uk/ukpga/2010/15/pdfs/ukpga_20100015_en.pdf (accessed 21 September 2020).

HM Government (2015a) *The Modern Slavery Act 2015*. Norwich: The Stationery Office. [online] Available at: www. legislation.gov.uk/ukpga/2015/30/pdfs/ukpga_20150030_en.pdf (accessed 21 September 2020).

HM Government (2015b) *The Serious Crime Act (2015)*. Norwich: The Stationery Office. [online] Available at: www. legislation.gov.uk/ukpga/2015/9/pdfs/ukpga_20150009_en.pdf (accessed 21 September 2020).

Home Office (2015a) *Controlling or Coercive Behaviour in an Intimate or Family Relationship: Statutory Guidance Framework*. London: Home Office. [online] Available at: https://assets.publishing.service.gov.uk/government/ uploads/system/uploads/attachment_data/file/482528/Controlling_or_coercive_behaviour_-_statutory_ guidance.pdf (accessed 21 September 2020).

Home Office (2015b) *Home Office Circular: Modern Slavery Act 2015*. London: Home Office. [online] Available at: https://assets.publishing.service.gov.uk/government/uploads/system/uploads/attachment_data/file/443797/ Circular_242015Final_1_.pdf (accessed 6 December 2020).

Home Office (2018) *Review of the Psychoactive Substances Act 2016*. London: APS Group on behalf of the Controller of Her Majesty's Stationery Office. [online] Available at: https://assets.publishing.service.gov.uk/government/ uploads/system/uploads/attachment_data/file/756896/Review_of_the_Psychoactive_Substances_Act__2016__ web_.pdf (accessed 21 September 2020).

House of Commons, Home Affairs Committee (2018) *Domestic Abuse: Ninth Report of Session 2017–2019*. [online] Available at: https://publications.parliament.uk/pa/cm201719/cmselect/cmhaff/1015/1015.pdf (accessed 21 September 2020).

Institute of Race Relations (IRR) (nd) *Definitions*. [online] Available at: www.irr.org.uk/research/statistics/ definitions (accessed 21 September 2020).

International Federation of Social Workers (IFSW) (2014) *Global Definition of Social Workers*. [online] Available at: www.ifsw.org/what-is-social-work/global-definition-of-social-work/ (accessed 21 September 2020).

Mir, G, Nocon, A and Ahmad, W (2001) *Learning Difficulties and Ethnicities*. London: Report to the Department of Health.

Munro, E (2010) *The Munro Review of Child Protection*. London: HM Government Department of Education.

Oliver, M (1983) *Social Work with Disabled People*. Basingstoke: Macmillan.

Oliver, M (1990) *The Politics of Disablement*. Basingstoke: Macmillan.

Oliver, M (2013) The Social Model of Disability: Thirty Years On. *Disability & Society*, 28(7): 1024–26.

Oshikanlu, R (2014) Rekindle Your Curiosity. *The Nursing Times*. [online] Available at: www.nursingtimes.net/ rekindle-your-curiosity/5070572.article (accessed 21 September 2020).

Rees, A, Agnew-Davies, R and Barkham, M (2006) *Outcomes for Women Escaping Domestic Violence at Refuge*. Paper presented at the Society for Psychotherapy Research Annual Conference, Edinburgh.

Rogers, C (1959) A Theory of Therapy, Personality and Interpersonal Relationships as Developed in the Client-centered Framework. In Koch, S (ed) *Psychology: A Study of a Science. Vol. 3: Formulations of the Person and the Social Context*. New York: McGraw Hill. [online] Available at: https://archive.org/stream/psychologyastudy017916mbp/ psychologyastudy017916mbp_djvu.txt (accessed 21 September 2020).

Stark, E (2007) *Coercive Control: How Men Entrap Women in Personal Life (Interpersonal Violence)*. New York, NY: Oxford University Press.

Stark, E (2009) Rethinking Coercive Control. *Violence Against Women*, 15: 1509–25.

Stark, E (2012) *Re-presenting Battered Women: Coercive Control and the Defence of Liberty*. Prepared for Violence Against Women: Complex Realities and New Issues in a Changing World, Les Presses de l'Université du Québec, Canada.

Stobart, E (2017) *Lessons Learnt from a Serious Case Review: BSCB 2016–17/1: 'I Just Wanted Someone To Ask Me' - Isobel*. Birmingham Safeguarding Children Board, UK. [online] Available at: www.lscpbirmingham.org.uk/ images/BSCP/Professionals/Serious_Case_Reviews/BSCP_17_01/Lessons_Learnt_from_a_Serious_Case_Review. pdf (accessed 21 September 2020).

Walklate, S, Fitz-Gibbon, K and McCulloch, J (2017) Is More Law the Answer? Seeking Justice for Victims of Intimate Partner Violence through Reform of Legal Categories. *Criminology & Criminal Justice*, 18(1): 115–31.

World Health Organization (WHO) (2018) *International Classification of Diseases - 11*. [online] Available at: www. who.int/classifications/icd/en/ (accessed 21 September 2020).

World Health Organization (WHO) (2019) *Management of Substance Abuse: Terminology and Classification.* [online] Available at: www.who.int/substance_abuse/terminology/psychoactive_substances/en/ (accessed 21 September 2020).

Publications

Clement, S (2011) Disability Hate Crime and Targeted Violence and Hostility: A Mental Health and Discrimination Perspective. *Journal of Mental Health*, 20(3): 219–25.

Johnson, K and Barlow, C (2018) *Researching Police Responses to Coercive Control.* Lancaster University: Policing Research Partnership. [online] Available at: https://n8prp.org.uk/researching-police-responses-to-coercive-control/ (accessed 21 September 2020).

Kuennen, T L (2007) Analyzing the Impact of Coercion on Domestic Violence Victims: How Much is Too Much. *Berkeley Journal of Gender, Law & Justice*, 22(2): Article 1. [online] Available at: https://doi.org/10.15779/Z38CR5NB8Q (accessed 21 September 2020).

Mir, G (2007) *Effective Communication with Service Users.* Better Health Briefing 2. London: Race Equality Foundation.

Oliver, M and Barnes, C (2012) *The New Politics of Disablement.* Basingstoke: Macmillan.

Pizzey, E (1979) *Scream Quietly or the Neighbours Will Hear.* London: Pelican.

Richardson, K and Fulton, R (2010) *Towards Culturally Competent Advocacy: Meeting the Needs of Diverse Communities.* Kidderminster: British Institute of Learning Disabilities (BILD). [online] Available at: www.gain.org.uk/documents/culturalcompetencypaper.pdf (accessed 21 September 2020).

Schechter, S (1982) *Women and Male Violence: The Visions and Struggles of the Battered Women's Movement.* Cambridge, MA: South End Press.

Schechter, S (1987) *Guidelines for Mental Health Practitioners in Domestic Violence Cases 4.* Denver, CO: National Coalition Against Domestic Violence.

Thomas, P (2011) 'Mate Crime': Ridicule, Hostility and Targeted Attacks Against Disabled People. *Disability & Society*, 26(1): 107–11.

Unwin, G, Larkin, M, Rose, J, Kroese, B S and Malcom, S (2016) Developing Resources to Facilitate Culturally-sensitive Service Planning and Delivery – Doing Research Inclusively with People with Learning Disabilities. *Research Involvement and Engagement*, 2: Article 17.

Websites

British Institute for Learning Disabilities: www.bild.org.uk (accessed 21 September 2020).

Disability Hate Crime: www.cps.gov.uk (accessed 21 September 2020).

Research in Practice for Adults: https://coercivecontrol.ripfa.org.uk (accessed 21 September 2020).

Women's Aid, UK: www.womensaid.org.uk/information-support (accessed 21 September 2020).

Introduction to the Social and Medical Models of Disability: www.ombudsman.org.uk/sites/default/files/FDN-218144_Introduction_to_the_Social_and_Medical_Models_of_Disability.pdf (accessed 21 September 2020).

Social Model of Disability: www.mentalhealth.org.uk/learning-disabilities/a-to-z/s/social-model-disability (accessed 21 September 2020).

Introduction

In our earlier work *Self-neglect: A Practical Approach to Risks and Strengths Assessment* (Britten and Whitby, 2018) we explained in detail a model risks and strengths intervention framework designed to support practitioners in consistent, clear and evidence-based practice. We do not intend here to replicate the complete toolkit of resources published previously; however, we have used this framework to demonstrate the adoption of MSP principles, as a practical approach to the Learning from Life case scenarios detailed in earlier chapters. Therefore, in this chapter, we have included a simplified overview graphic of the process, with descriptive prompts included as illustrative risks and strengths assessments based upon the Learning from Life examples.

Also included within this chapter is discussion and description of the need for practitioners to establish and maintain their legal literacy in key areas of legislation and common law in England, the principles of which can hold relevance in other jurisdictions with differing legislative systems. Also raised are the tensions which can exist between the impotence or refusal of some individuals to manage their own personal health, well-being and safety in relation to their own potential demotivation or impotence to effect change.

Included in this chapter are *SnapShots on...* practice resources, designed to expand upon and summarise some factors of relevance to the Learning from Life case scenarios, and as aids to prompt further exploration by practitioners; these topic areas are:

» Attachment.

» The 'toxic trio'.

» Adverse childhood experiences (ACEs).

Taking a 'risks and strengths balance' (Figure 3.1) approach to assessment enables:

» the person to be placed at the centre and in control (based upon individual needs, circumstances and legal requirements);

» an evaluation of potential and/or actual risk factors;

» the identification of personal and/or social strengths which mitigate those risks.

Figure 3.1 Living life is not risk-free!

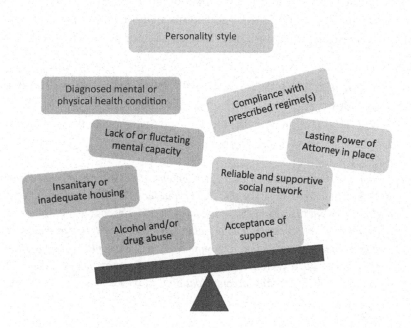

In Chapter 2, we discussed the adoption of active listening skills during conversations in practice as an effective means to establish and maintain a relationship based upon empathy, unconditional positive regard and genuineness (Rogers, 1959). In progressing a risks and strengths assessment, active and reflective listening skills remain of vital importance in establishing the personal and/or social strengths available to an individual which mitigate actual or potential risks of harm or neglect.

Legal literacy

Taking risks in life is a basic human right and must be respected and promoted throughout all conversations, assessment and protection planning in safeguarding. All practitioners should promote and continually develop their own legal literacy as a means to remain fully aware of the legislative and legal frameworks within which they practice and awareness of when they may need to seek specific legal advice from a lawyer/solicitor, within their line management structure and organisational arrangements. This level of knowledge and insight is of particular importance in the context of risk, rights and responsibilities – fundamental components of empowerment and self-determination. A selection of key pieces of UK law and legislative issues are included below. The legal duties and powers enshrined within the Care Act (2014) and the Mental Capacity Act (2005) are well-known and clearly documented in many texts, and therefore have not been included here specifically other than in consideration of fluctuations in a person's mental capacity to make a decision at the time it needs to be made (see 'Cognitive fluctuations, demotivation or impotence', below) – this is not an unconscious omission, more a pragmatic approach to avoid unnecessary duplication.

The Deprivation of Liberty Safeguards (DoLS) 2007 (Ministry of Justice, 2008) and subsequent case law include the Supreme Court Judgment in the UK (often referred to as 'Cheshire West') where Lady Hale (Judge and President of the Supreme Court) famously stated '*A gilded cage is still a cage*' when delivering judgment in the case:

In my view, it is axiomatic that people with disabilities, both mental and physical, have the same human rights as the rest of the human race. It may be that those rights have sometimes to be limited or restricted because of their disabilities, but the starting point should be the same as that for everyone else. This flows inexorably from the universal character of human rights, founded on the inherent dignity of all human beings, and is confirmed in the United Nations Convention on the Rights of Persons with Disabilities. Far from disability entitling the state to deny such people human rights: rather it places upon the state (and upon others) the duty to make reasonable accommodation to cater for the special needs of those with disabilities.

(Supreme Court, 2014)

In addition, practitioners should ensure that they are familiar and competent to progress applications to the Court of Protection under the procedure known as 'Re X' (Court of Appeal, 2015). This relates to any circumstances or settings where the DoLS application process in Schedule A1 (hospital and care home residents) of the Mental Capacity Act (2005) cannot be used; and also where the person is between the age of 16 and 18.

At the time of writing, confirmation remains awaited regarding the passing into law and implementation of a scheme referred to as 'Liberty Protection Safeguards' in the UK, in replacement of DoLS.

Of particular note in relation to the adoption of an MSP approach in risks and strengths assessment, the following Articles of the Human Rights Act (1998) should be adhered to in any/all casework:

ARTICLE 2 Right to Life

Everyone's right to life must be protected by law. There are only extremely limited circumstances where it is legally acceptable for the State to use force against a person that results in their death, for example, a Police Officer can use reasonable force to defend themselves or to protect other people.

ARTICLE 3 Prohibition of Torture

Everyone has the absolute right to be free of torture or to be subjected to treatment or punishment that is inhuman and/or degrading.

ARTICLE 4 Right to Liberty and Security

Everyone has the right not to be deprived of their liberty, except in limited cases specified within the Article, for example where they are suspected or convicted of committing a crime, and provided there is a proper legal basis in UK law for their arrest or detention.

ARTICLE 6 Right to a Fair Trial

Everyone has the right to a fair and public hearing, within a reasonable period of time. This applies to both criminal charges being brought, and in cases concerning civil rights and obligations. According to the law, a person who is charged with an offence is presumed innocent until proven guilty, and must also be guaranteed certain minimum rights in relation to the conduct of the criminal investigation and trial.

ARTICLE 8 Right to Respect for Private and Family Life

Everyone has the right to respect for their private and family life; their home and their correspondence; 'There shall be no interference by a public authority with the exercise of this right except such as is in accordance with the law and is necessary in a democratic society in the interests of national security, public safety or the economic well-being of the country, for the prevention of disorder or crime, for the protection of health or morals, or for the protection of the rights and freedoms of others.'

The European Court of Human Rights knowledge and application of the law has determined that private life covers 'a person's physical and psychological integrity', 'personal development', and 'personal autonomy'. The court has also interpreted this right to protect people from the 'disruption of home or family life' causing 'stress and distress'.

ARTICLE 14 Prohibition of Discrimination

In the application of all other convention rights, people have the right to not be treated differently because of their race, religion, gender, political views or any other protected characteristics unless there is an 'objective justification' for the difference.

(HM Government, 1998)

Examples of other legislation of relevance in safeguarding include (not exhaustive):

Offences Against the Person Act	1861
Theft Act	1968
Mental Health Act	1983
Police and Criminal Evidence Act	1984
Criminal Justice Act	1988
Protection from Harassment Act	1997
The Crime and Disorder Act	1998
Youth Justice and Criminal Evidence Act	1999
Sexual Offences Act	2003
Criminal Justice Act	2003
Domestic Violence and Criminal Evidence Act	2004
Equalities Act	2010
The Modern Slavery Act	2015
Serious Crime Act	2015
The Psychoactive Substances Act	2016

Of particular note for practitioners to explore further is the legal requirement for support to be offered and made available to those people who are 'vulnerable witnesses' in criminal proceedings such as giving evidence in a criminal investigation by the police and if/when they are required to appear in court. The Youth and Criminal Evidence Act (1999) Section 16, defines a 'vulnerable witness' as:

1) *For the purposes of this Chapter a witness in criminal proceedings (other than the accused) is eligible for assistance by virtue of this section –*

   (a) *if under the age of 17 at the time of the hearing; or*
   (b) *if the court considers that the quality of evidence given by the witness is likely to be diminished by reason of any circumstances falling within subsection (2).*

2) *The circumstances falling within this subsection are –*

   (a) *that the witness –*
      i. *suffers from mental disorder within the meaning of the Mental Health Act 1983, or 1983 c. 20.*
      ii. *otherwise has a significant impairment of intelligence and social functioning;*
   (b) *that the witness has a physical disability or is suffering from a physical disorder.*

Some disabilities are obvious, some are hidden. Witnesses may have a combination of disabilities. They may not wish to disclose the fact that they have a disability during initial and subsequent needs assessments. Different witnesses on the autistic spectrum may have very different needs.

(HM Government, 1999, Section 16)

Cognitive fluctuations, demotivation or impotence

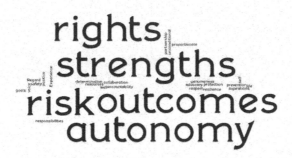

In expanding upon accurate risks and strengths assessment, consideration should be given to whether a person is making an unwise decision or if they may be experiencing fluctuations in their mental capacity to make a specific decision at the time it needs to be made. In cases where there are queries or concerns about a person's mental capacity, an assessment should be undertaken and recorded. This is discussed in Chapter 2, '*SnapShot on...* the Mental Capacity Act (2005) and best interests decision-making'.

The area of fluctuating capacity and motivation can be described as a tension between the impotence and refusal of some individuals to manage their own personal health, well-being and safety; in simple terms, as 'cognitive stuckness', a concept identified by consultant psychiatrist Dr Andrew Heighton (MBChB, MRCPsych). This state of cognitive fluctuation (Figure 3.2) can expand or contract based upon a spectrum of strengths, resilience, and pressures (push and pull factors), such as:

» pressure from external bodies or agencies (for example Environmental Health, a landlord, the police, or the perceptions of local neighbours, family or community who apply pressure to local services to intervene);

» peer, parental or familial support provision or withdrawal;

» changes or fluctuations in mental or physical health;

» coercion;

» alcohol or drug abuse;

» perceptions of threat, and the potential triggering of survival behaviours;

» personality and thinking styles.

Figure 3.2 A state of cognitive fluctuation

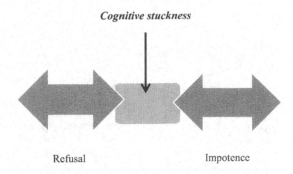

Cognitive stuckness

Refusal   Impotence

In the context of the tension described above, there is also a need to consider any physical health diagnosis which may in the future have an impact upon the person's ability to care for themselves and/or their home environment. The cumulative total of 'refusal' (both historic and current) and the potential future 'impotence' of the individual needs to be considered from a preventative perspective in order to mitigate the risk of an escalation of concerns and must be included within any protection planning process.

Supporting a person with care and support needs who has experienced harm or neglect is a highly complex human event, even when the circumstances may appear to be straightforward. People in these situations may have a reduced capacity to tolerate change and may have developed unhelpful survival behaviours. This presentation has been described by Dr Andrew Heighton as *'driving and restraining forces – a human perspective'*; included in Chapter 5 is information adapted, with his permission, from a presentation he gave in September 2017.

A risks and strengths assessment model framework

The following flowchart (Figure 3.3) is adapted from the model outlined in more detail in our earlier publication (Britten and Whitby, 2018) as a visual representation of safeguarding risks and strengths assessment and protection planning.

Figure 3.3 Model framework for risks and strengths assessment

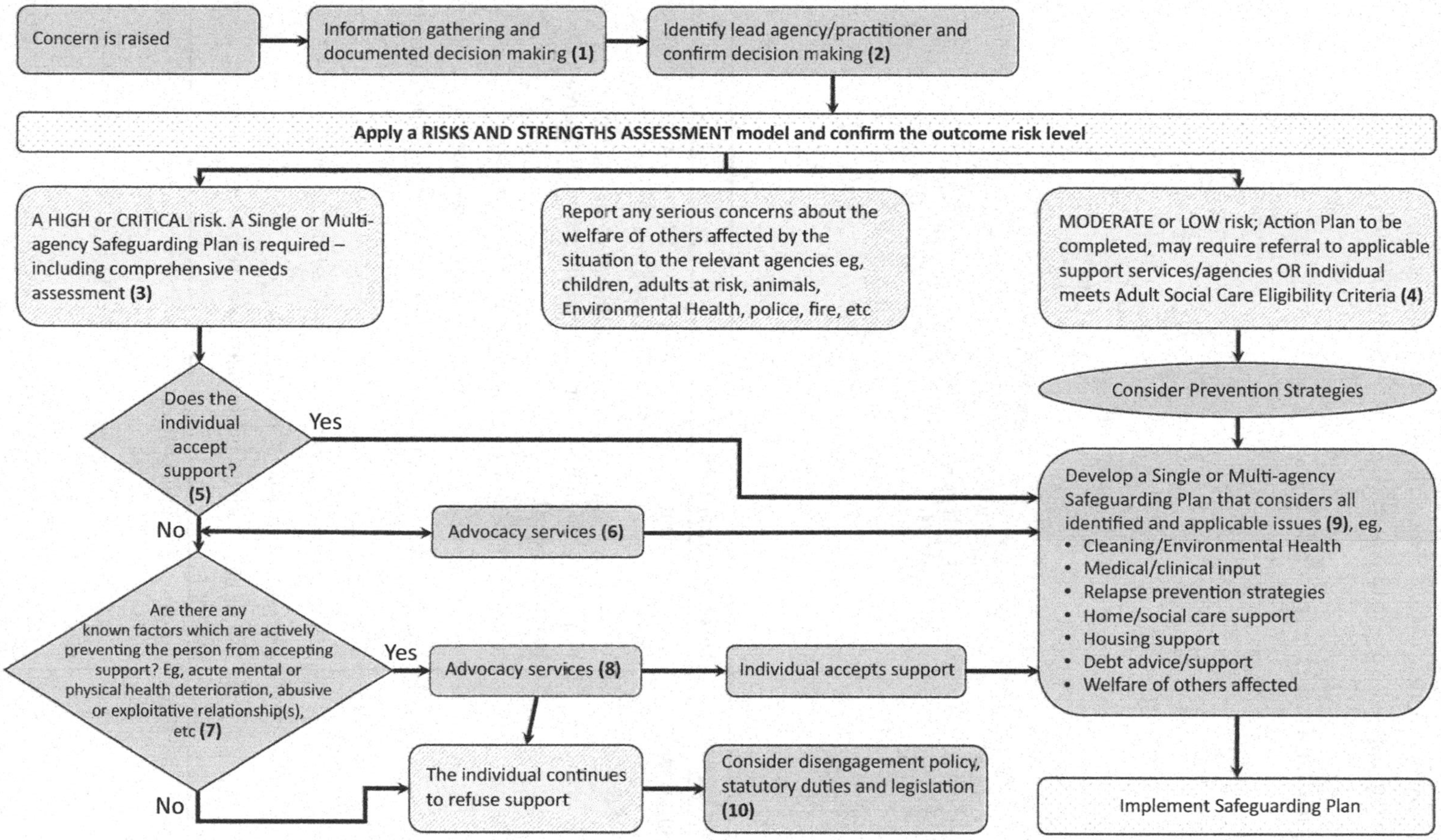

In approaching risks and strengths assessment, and as a means to achieve clarity and consistency in practice, we use a set of 'key factors' and associated prompts, as the basis from which to begin the evaluation of risks and personal/social strengths (Figure 3.4).

Figure 3.4 Factors in self-neglect

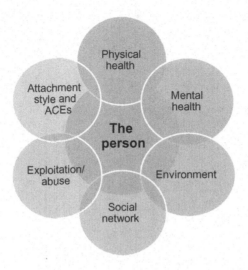

Key factor	Description/prompts
Mental health	Diagnosed mental health condition, learning disability/difficulties and/or impaired cognition, including Diogenes Syndrome.
	A recent deterioration in mental health state (may include the lack of motivation to meet essential personal care needs, recent loss/bereavement and/or traumatic event).
	Involvement with specialist healthcare professionals.
	Non-concordance with treatment plan and/or prescribed medication regime.
	Lack of or fluctuating mental capacity to make informed decisions in this regard, following assessment in line with the requirements of the Mental Capacity Act (2005).
	Known pattern of problematic alcohol use/dependency.
	Known pattern of illegal substance misuse.
	Involvement with the police and/or probation service (may include MAPPA/ MARAC).
Physical health	Recognised 'long-term/enduring condition' for which treatment/medicine is prescribed.
	'Long-term/enduring condition' which has the potential to reduce life expectancy if not managed.
	Deterioration in physical health state and/or exacerbation of an existing condition.

Key factor	Description/prompts
	Involvement with specialist healthcare professionals.
	Non-concordance with treatment plan and/or prescribed medication regime.
	Non-secure tenure – may be assured shorthold *or* informal arrangement (this can include, for example, bed-and-breakfast accommodation and/or 'sofa-surfing').
	Not suitable to meet needs – mobility or environmental factors.
Environment and housing	Inadequate essential amenities (utilities).
	Refusal to engage with support agencies.
	Unsanitary conditions and/or hoarding (objects and/or animals) which will lead to the involvement of Environmental Health services and may also include fire services.
Social network and lifestyle choices	Relationships – which may be problematic, hazardous and/or abusive (including alcohol/substance dependencies).
	Children and/or other adults at risk living at the property.
	Limited/no reliable social network of family/friends *and/or* risks posed by a carer.
	Known pattern of involvement with the criminal justice system.
	Known pattern of involvement with statutory agencies (including crisis intervention).
	Homelessness.
	Debt with inadequate resources to meet demands.
	Involvement with the police and/or probation service (may include MAPPA/MARAC).
	Young adults at risk in transition from children to adult social care services.
Exploitation/ abuse	Involvement with statutory agencies regarding allegations of abuse (in line with safeguarding adults definition).
	Known involvement with criminal justice offenders and/or perpetrators of abuse.
	Low self-esteem/worth.
	'Attention-seeking' behaviours which are potentially hazardous (eg, attachment disorders).
	Changes in usual routines, refusal to discuss the basis or nature of these changes.
	Deterioration in 'usual' personal presentation; this may include physical signs of assault and/or withdrawal from engagement/involvement.
	Involvement with the police and/or probation service (may include MAPPA/MARAC).
	Young adults at risk in transition from children to adult social care services.

Key factor	Description/prompts
Attachment style and early life experiences	Early life trauma (adverse childhood experiences) including: • neglect – failure to thrive; • physical abuse; • emotional abuse; • 'toxic trio' within the family unit; • sexual abuse; • self-blame; • self-harm; • inability to maintain healthy attachment relationship with parent or primary caregiver.

Other factors for practitioners to consider/evaluate in particular circumstances include responsibilities to maintain the reputation of their profession and organisation/agency from adverse publicity and/or damage.

Adverse publicity	Rumours; potential for public concern. Local, short-term media coverage – minimal public concern.
Damage to the reputation of the agency and public confidence	Local media-coverage – long-term reduction in public confidence. National media coverage – long-term reduction in public confidence. National media coverage which includes the attention of the local parliamentary representative and a total loss of public confidence. A complaint which may include referral and/or investigation by the Ombudsman. Criteria for a Safeguarding Adults Review may be met. Potential for litigation; criminal prosecution. Breach(es) in statutory duty (including the duty of candour). MAPPA arrangements.

Learning from Life case scenarios

A risks and strengths assessment (Britten and Whitby, 2018) approach was adopted to build a clear and evidenced-based picture of each of the case scenarios using the key factors to describe presenting risk factors and calculate risk levels; these are summarised below.

This initial analysis was then balanced with the incorporation of the individual's strengths and agreed actions to be taken to mitigate the impact and likelihood of the harm or neglect from occurring; example protection plans are included in Chapter 4.

Scenario one – JA

Key factor	Description/prompts
Mental health Impact = 5 Likelihood = 5 Outcome = 25 CRITICAL IMMEDIATE	Diagnosed mental health conditions: schizophrenia, obsessive compulsive disorder (OCD), '6A02.0 Autism spectrum disorder without disorder of intellectual development and with mild or no impairment of functional language' (WHO, 2018).
	'Linear' interpretation/communication – unable to engage in abstract or seemingly unconnected conversations without pictorial aids, and careful construction of sentences (knowledge and skill is required to minimise misunderstandings and agitation).
	A recent deterioration in mental health well-being, including the lack of ability/motivation to meet essential personal care needs, 'cognitive stuckness', increased anxiety.
	Involvement with community mental healthcare professionals.
	Non-concordance with treatment plan and/or prescribed medication regime – history of overdose, suicidal ideology, invasive thoughts.
	Fluctuating mental capacity to make specific, informed decisions at the time they need to be made, following an assessment in line with the requirements of the Mental Capacity Act (2005).
	Historical pattern of involvement with the police (Section 136 of the Mental Health Act (1983); used to take him to a place of safety on numerous occasions.
Physical health Impact = 3 Likelihood = 5 Outcome = 15 CRITICAL IMMEDIATE	Deterioration in physical health state: extreme oral decay, hair loss, severe deterioration in sight.
	Intolerance of everyday sounds – interplay/impact upon mental health well-being.
	Non-concordance with treatment plan and/or prescribed medication regime.
Environment and housing Impact = 4 Likelihood = 5 Outcome = 20 CRITICAL IMMEDIATE	Tenancy under threat due to extreme clutter and insanitary conditions.
	Inadequate essential amenities (utilities).
	Refusal/impotence to engage with support agencies, 'cognitive stuckness'.
	Involvement of Environmental Health Services and Fire and Rescue Services.
Social network and lifestyle choices Impact = 2 Likelihood = 3 Outcome = 6 MODERATE	Unreliable social relationships – described (not evidenced) victim of 'doorstep scams' and 'friends' who may/may not have removed possessions from the property ('mate crime').
	Limited family support – mother is frail and lives some distance away, sibling is not involved.

Key factor	Description/prompts
Exploitation/abuse Impact = 4 Likelihood = 3 Outcome = 12 HIGH	Involvement with statutory agencies regarding allegations of abuse – reported verbally abusive behaviour by a neighbour, concerns of self-neglect reported to Environmental Health. Has a sense of low self-worth; will quickly build relationships of trust with people he immediately regards as friends (see 'social network' factor above). Deterioration in 'usual' personal presentation ('cognitive stuckness').
Attachment style and early life experiences Impact = 1 Likelihood = 1 Outcome = 2 LOW	Reported 'toxic trio' within the family unit; no formal details.
Adverse publicity damage to the reputation of the agency and public confidence Impact = 3 Likelihood = 3 Outcome = 9 HIGH	Rumours; potential for public concern. Potential for local media coverage. The local MP is aware. A complaint which may include referral and/or investigation by the Ombudsman. Criteria for a Safeguarding Adults Review may be met. Breach(es) in statutory duty.

Scenario two – CD

As noted above, a risks and strengths assessment (Britten and Whitby, 2018) approach was adopted to build a clear and evidenced-based picture of presenting risk factors. This initial analysis was then balanced with the incorporation of the individual's strengths and agreed actions to be taken to mitigate the impact and likelihood of the harm or neglect occurring; the example protection plan is included in Chapter 4.

Initial risk levels are summarised below.

Key factor	Description/prompts
Mental health Impact = 5 Likelihood = 5 Outcome = 25 CRITICAL IMMEDIATE	Diagnosed paranoid schizophrenia, personality disorder, learning difficulty. A recent deterioration in mental health well-being; serious self-harming/cutting behaviours. Involvement with community mental healthcare professionals. Non-concordance with treatment plan and/or prescribed medication regime. History of involvement with the police under Section 136 of the Mental Health Act (1983) to take her to a place of safety.

Key factor	Description/prompts
Physical health Impact = 4 Likelihood = 4 Outcome = 16 HIGH	Tablet controlled diabetes, sleep apnoea and morbid obesity, which have the potential to reduce life expectancy if not managed. Self-harm/cutting injuries which require assessment and dressing by community-based nurses. Involvement with community nursing service. Current non-concordance with treatment plan: removing dressings and picking cuts open.
Environment and housing Impact = 4 Likelihood = 3 Outcome = 12 HIGH	Maintenance of specialist housing provision with ongoing support.
Social network and lifestyle choices Impact = 2 Likelihood = 3 Outcome = 6 MODERATE	Social isolation. No reliable social network of family/friends – reliant upon support staff for social interactions. Known pattern of involvement with statutory agencies (including crisis intervention).
Exploitation/abuse Impact = 5 Likelihood = 5 Outcome = 25 CRITICAL IMMEDIATE	Involvement with statutory agencies regarding allegations of abuse; previous allegations of physical and sexual assault (rape) not progressed as criminal investigations or prosecutions. Known historic involvement with criminal justice offenders and perpetrators of abuse. Low self-esteem/worth. 'Attention-seeking' behaviours which are potentially hazardous (including and linked with attachment disorder and adverse ACEs – see below).
Attachment style and early life experiences Impact = 5 Likelihood = 5 Outcome = 25 CRITICAL IMMEDIATE	Early life trauma (adverse childhood experiences) which have continuing impacts in adulthood; these include: • neglect – failure to thrive; • physical abuse; • emotional abuse; • 'toxic trio' within the family unit; • sexual abuse; • self-blame; • self-harm; • inability to maintain healthy attachment relationship with parent or primary caregiver.

Adverse publicity damage to the reputation of the agency and public confidence	Rumours; potential for public concern.
Impact = 1	
Likelihood = 2	
Outcome = 2 LOW	

Practice matters

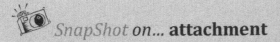 *SnapShot* on... **attachment**

This *SnapShot* is designed to give practitioners a practical overview of the complex and much-researched issue of attachment in early life, and its potential implications in adulthood as a consideration in safeguarding; it aims to prompt and actively encourage more detailed exploration of this complex subject area. It is divided under two headings.

» An overview of 'attachment theory'.

» Safeguarding adults and risk factors.

An overview of 'attachment theory'

The theory of attachment and its association with personality development was first proposed by John Bowlby (British psychologist and psychoanalyst) in the mid-twentieth century; he is well known for the description of attachment, frequently attributed to him, as a *'lasting psychological connectedness between human beings'*. Bowlby expanded understanding and acceptance of the concept that early life experiences can have an impact *'on how someone's personality has come to be structured turns his way of responding to subsequent adverse events, among which rejections, separations, and losses are some of the most important'* (Bowlby, 1982 [1969], p 300).

Bowlby considered that in order to grow and develop positively in both mental and emotional health through their lifespan, children needed to develop a secure attachment with their main caregiver in their early years:

what is believed to be essential for mental health is that the infant and young child should experience a warm, intimate, and continuous relationship with his mother (or permanent mother substitute) in which both find satisfaction and enjoyment.

(Bowlby, 1952, p 11)

It is important to note that the early focus (recognising the language and perceptions of the time) was not purely placed upon a natural/birth mother, but also on a *'perma-nent mother substitute'*, later referred to as an attachment figure:

Bowlby, after all, was careful to use the term attachment figure rather than mother, because of his belief that, although biological mothers typically serve as principal attachment figures, other figures such as fathers, adoptive mothers, grandparents, and childcare providers can also serve as attachment figures.

(Cassidy et al, 2013)

During his career, Bowlby worked collaboratively with Mary Ainsworth, an American-born psychologist, and founded concepts of attachment which remain referenced and used to this day.

Ainsworth undertook the extensive observational study of interactions between mothers and their infants published as a journal article in *Child Development*: 'Attachment, Exploration, and Separation: Illustrated by the Behavior of One-Year-Olds in a Strange Situation' (Ainsworth and Bell, 1970). The outcome of this work formed the basis for what is now referred to as the 'Strange Situation Procedure'; in brief this involved observations of an infant's reactions to eight situations, each lasting a few minutes.

1. Mother, infant and observer together.

2. Mother and infant alone.

3. A stranger joins the mother and infant.

4. Mother leaves the infant and stranger alone.

5. Mother returns and the stranger leaves.

6. Mother leaves and the infant is alone.

7. The stranger returns to join the infant.

8. Mother returns and the stranger leaves.

The behaviours/reactions shown by the infant to the mother, when she returned, were recorded using four measures.

1. Seeking contact with the mother.

2. Maintaining contact with the mother.

3. Avoidance of contact with the mother.

4. Resistance to contact with the mother.

Further comprehensive scientific evaluation of the data gathered identified three attachment forms/types which were described as: secure, insecure avoidant and insecure ambivalent/resistant.

An extremely useful paper for practitioners looking for more information about the origins of John Bowlby's and Mary Ainsworth's works was published by Inge Bretherton in 1992, *The Origins of Attachment Theory: John Bowlby and Mary Ainsworth*. In this paper, Bretherton acknowledges both Mary Ainsworth and Ursula Bowlby *'for helpful input on a draft of this article'*. Full details of how to find this resource and others are included in the *Taking It Further* section at the end of this chapter.

Since this time, a multitude of further studies have expanded the understanding and definition of attachment types, with formally diagnosed conditions contained within the *International Classification of Diseases – 11* (WHO, 2018) as:

6B44 Reactive attachment disorder

Reactive attachment disorder is characterized by grossly abnormal attachment behaviours in early childhood, occurring in the context of a history of grossly inadequate childcare (eg, severe neglect, maltreatment, institutional deprivation). Even when an adequate primary caregiver is newly available, the child does not turn to the primary caregiver for comfort, support and nurture, rarely displays security-seeking behaviours towards any adult, and does not respond when comfort is offered. Reactive attachment disorder can only be diagnosed in children, and features of the disorder develop within the first 5 years of life. However, the disorder cannot be diagnosed before the age of 1 year (or a developmental age of less than 9 months), when the capacity for selective attachments may not be fully developed, or in the context of Autism spectrum disorder.

6B45 Disinhibited social engagement disorder

Disinhibited social engagement disorder is characterized by grossly abnormal social behaviour, occurring in the context of a history of grossly inadequate childcare (eg, severe neglect, institutional deprivation). The child approaches adults indiscriminately, lacks reticence to approach, will go away with unfamiliar adults, and exhibits overly familiar behaviour towards strangers. Disinhibited social engagement disorder can only be diagnosed in children, and features of the disorder develop within the first 5 years of life. However, the disorder cannot be diagnosed before the age of 1 year (or a developmental age of less than 9 months), when the capacity for selective attachments may not be fully developed, or in the context of Autism spectrum disorder.

In practical terms attachment can be summarised as 'secure' or 'insecure':

Secure attachments support mental processes that enable the individual to regulate emotions, reduce fear, build relationships with others, have self-awareness, empathy and understanding, and importantly, build internal/personal resilience to support effective decision-making factors. Bowlby (1973) referred to these factors as the *'Internal Working Model'*.

Insecure attachments can have unfortunate consequences if the child cannot rely upon the primary caregiver to respond to their needs in times of stress; they can become unable to soothe/reassure themselves to manage their emotions and response, and in some cases to engage in positive reciprocal relationships. Where the child's experiences in early life and their dependencies on their primary caregiver for soothing protection and positive interactions (their Internal Working Model, referred to above) have not been met, the insecurities, lack of self-confidence, stress and fear experienced can result in inabilities to establish or maintain positive relationships in adulthood. The 'insecure' attachment is categorised as either:

> **'Ambivalent'** where the person has experienced unpredictable and inconsistent caregiving – this can present itself as 'seeking' security, comfort, and care but then being unable to accept it being available. This form of attachment can also be associated with people who may appear to be immature, attention-seeking, hyperactive, fussy, helpless or passive, and the opposite as angry and petulant individuals.

> **'Avoidant'** where the person has experienced the absence and/or rejection from their primary caregiver when they have sought security, comfort and care from them. This form of attachment can be associated with people who are task-orientated and self-sufficient in life, but who can also show indifference, an inability to feel/show empathy to others and have difficulty forming positive close personal relationships. They may also have difficulty in asking for or accepting help/assistance, and could be prone to sudden angry outbursts.

Adult attachment theorists (eg, Collins & Read, 1994; Dykas & Cassidy, 2011; Shaver, Collins & Clark, 1996) view working models as cognitive-affective structures that include autobiographical, episodic memories (concrete memories of specific interactions with attachment figures), beliefs concerning oneself and relationship partners, declarative knowledge about attachment relationships and interactions (eg, the belief that romantic love as portrayed in movies does not exist in real life), and procedural knowledge about how to regulate emotions and behave in close relationships.

(Mikulincer and Shaver, 2016 [2007], p 21)

In the 1980s an approach to the assessment of experiences of attachment with a parent/primary caregiver in early life began development in order to identify if those experiences had had an impact on the adult; this is called the Adult Attachment Interview (AAI) (George et al, 1985). The AAI is a set of open questions about an individual adult's memories of their childhood relationship with their parent/primary caregiver, with the outcome evaluation categories similar to the forms of attachment originally identified by Mary Ainsworth in her earlier works: secure, dismissive, preoccupied. The details and evaluation of this assessment process and the impacts of attachment in adulthood are discussed by Mikulincer and Shaver (2016 [2007]) in an accessible and very readable format – we would highly recommend this as a valuable addition to any practitioner's bookshelf; details are included within the *Taking It Further* section at the end of this chapter.

Ongoing extensive research and insightful learning for all practitioners includes the works of Dr Bruce D Perry, a leading psychiatrist, researcher and author of the impacts of cognitive, behavioural, emotional, social and physiological neglect and trauma in children, adolescents and adults; he expands attachment to encompass the concept of 'human relationships'. In the introduction to his book *The Boy Who Was Raised as a Dog*, Perry describes

I have long been interested in understanding human development, especially in trying to figure out why some people grow up to be productive, responsible, and kind human beings, whereas others respond to abuse by inflicting more of it on others. My work has revealed to me a great deal about moral development, about the roots of evil and how genetic tendencies and environmental influences can shape critical decisions, which in turn affect later choices, and ultimately, who we turn out to be. I do not believe in 'the abuse excuse' for violent or hurtful behavior, but I have found that there are complex interactions beginning in early childhood that affect our ability to envision choices and that may later limit our ability to make the best decisions.

(Perry and Szalavitz, 2006, p xxviii)

Safeguarding adults and risk factors

The originating theory base of 'attachment' and its impacts upon personality development has further expanded to identify that multiple attachments can occur throughout the lifespan (for example, in romantic relationships), and that early life experiences may continue to have an impact into adulthood. *'What began as a theory of child development is now used to conceptualize and study adult couple relationships, work relationships, and relations between social groups and societies'* (Mikulincer and Shaver, 2016 [2007], p 4). In their publication *Attachment in Adulthood: Structure, Dynamics, and Change* (2016 [2007]), Mikulincer and Shaver explore and detail associations between 'anxious' and 'avoidant' attachment types and the increased risk of violence in adulthood both as the source of harm and as the 'victim'.

In approaching a Safeguarding Adults Enquiry consideration should be given to whether attachment experiences in childhood and earlier life may predispose or have an impact upon the resilience of the individual to make choices and decisions in relation to the risk posed. Key issues to be considered at the start of a Safeguarding Adults Enquiry are shown in Figure 3.5.

Figure 3.5 Considering earlier life experiences

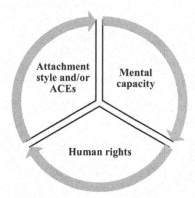

In our earlier work *Self-neglect: A Practical Approach to Risk and Strengths Assessment* (Britten and Whitby, 2018), we suggest the lifespan of trauma in childhood, the potential development of attachment disorder, and the impact of puberty, interpersonal relationships and pressures be considered as potential risk factors for the manifestation of self-neglecting behaviours in adulthood for some people, while fully recognising that this isn't always the case.

Factors for consideration are included within Figure 3.6, including early life trauma (ACEs, described in the *SnapShot on...* included below) such as:

» neglect – failure to thrive;

» physical abuse;

» emotional abuse;

» 'toxic trio' within the family unit;

» sexual abuse;

» self-blame;

» self-harm;

» inability to maintain healthy attachment relationship with parent or primary caregiver;

» 'attention seeking' behaviours which are potentially hazardous.

Figure 3.6 A spectrum of risk

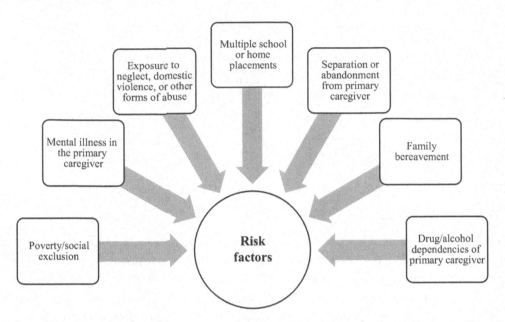

People vulnerable to the impacts, in their adult life, of insecure attachment can include, for example:

» a childhood growing up in areas of social and economic deprivation;

» institutional care arrangements during childhood;

» adopted children whose early life trauma continues to affect their lives;

» refugees who have experienced the trauma of war, conflict and loss;

» those with medical conditions such as post-traumatic stress disorder (PTSD).

SnapShot on... **the 'toxic trio'**

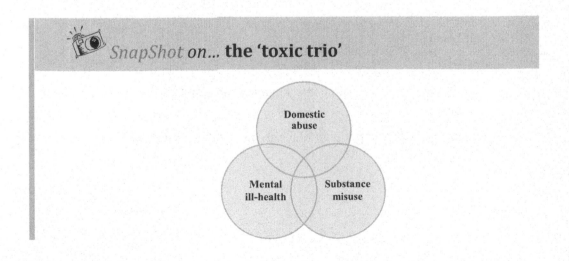

This *SnapShot* is designed to give practitioners an overview of the term 'toxic trio', which has been used to describe the combined impact of the issues of domestic abuse, mental ill-health and substance misuse that have been identified as a common feature where harm to children or adults at risk has occurred.

The 'toxic trio' are indicators of increased risk to families and are significant factors in interpersonal violence (IPV) and adult family violence (AFV).

Definitions

» The Home Office definition of *domestic violence and abuse* (Strickland and Allen, 2018) includes any incident or pattern of incidents of controlling, coercive or threatening behaviour or violence between those aged 16 or over who are or have been intimate partners or family members regardless of gender or sexuality.

» *Working our Way to Better Mental Health: A Framework for Action* (Department for Work and Pensions and the Department of Health, 2009, p 11) describes the wide range of conditions covered by the term *mental ill health*, including depression, anxiety and psychotic illnesses such as schizophrenia or bipolar disorder. Mental illness may also be associated with alcohol or drug use, personality disorder and significant physical illness.

» The National Institute for Health and Care Excellence (NICE) Quality Standard 23 states: '*Drug use disorders are defined as intoxication by, dependence on, or regular, excessive consumption of psychoactive substances leading to social, psychological, physical or legal problems*' (NICE, 2012, p 6). It includes the problematic use of both legal and illegal drugs (including alcohol when used in combination with other substances).

Why it matters

The 'toxic trio' are viewed as indicators of increased risk of harm to children, young people and increasingly to adults at risk (as defined by the Care Act 2014) and are common features where harm has occurred. An analysis of Child Practice Reviews undertaken by the North Wales Safeguarding Board showed that in

86% [of cases] where children were seriously harmed or died one or more of the 'toxic trio' played a significant part. Nearly two-thirds of these cases featured domestic abuse and in 60% mental ill-health was identified in one or both parents. Children in one-quarter of the families experienced all three. The effects on children often include poor attachment, poor school attendance, babies failing to thrive, low self esteem and other signs of neglect including being unkempt and looking uncared for.

(NWSB, 2017, np)

Children are exposed to significant risks and the harmful effects can be long-term and corrosive and have far-reaching implications into adulthood. Work in this area has demonstrated that there is an overlap between these parental risk factors and the potential impact on outcomes for children lasting into their adulthood through research into adverse childhood experience:

A growing body of research identifies the harmful effects that adverse childhood experiences (ACEs; occurring during childhood or adolescence; eg, child maltreatment or exposure to domestic violence) have on health throughout life. Studies have quantified such effects for individual ACEs.

(Hughes et al, 2017, p 356)

What should practitioners do and be aware of?

» Make sure that any immediate harm is managed – ensuring the safety of children or adults at risk is paramount.

» Know how to identify the common signs of abuse and neglect, who to escalate the issue to and how to refer to both children's and adult social care agencies.

The authors suggest that mandatory safeguarding training sessions should include awareness-raising and information in relation to the 'toxic trio'.

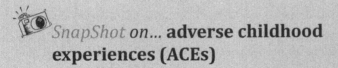 *SnapShot on...* **adverse childhood experiences (ACEs)**

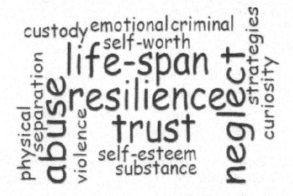

This *SnapShot* aims to:

» explain what adverse childhood experiences (ACEs) can be;

» highlight what is known about the extent and impact of the issues raised;

» outline some examples of what is known that may help in the prevention of ACEs and ameliorate the impact.

What are ACEs and what problems can they cause?

Adverse childhood experiences are traumatic events that have occurred to an individual before they have reached the age of 18 years.

There is now emerging a robust evidence base that links ACEs to what can be severe negative health and social care outcomes into adulthood and across the lifespan, including the leading causes of illness and death in the UK. This evidence base initially came from large population studies in the United States of America (Felitti et al, 1998), which have been replicated in studies undertaken worldwide including England (Bellis et al, 2014) and Wales (Ashton et al, 2016).

Research has defined ten factors which can be linked to ACEs; five directly relate to the child (Figure 3.7) and five relate to the parent/household (Figure 3.8). Exposure to a combination of these ten factors has been identified, by the Centers for Disease Control and Prevention (CDC, 2014), as linked with an increased risk of poor physical and/or mental health in the later life. These health conditions have been identified to include cancer, heart disease, diabetes, depression and anxiety as well as negative social outcomes such as domestic violence, low levels of educational achievement, criminal activity resulting in custodial sentences, and ultimately early death when compared to people who have had no exposure to ACEs.

Figure 3.7 ACE factors – child

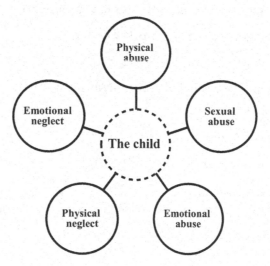

Figure 3.8 ACE factors – parent/household

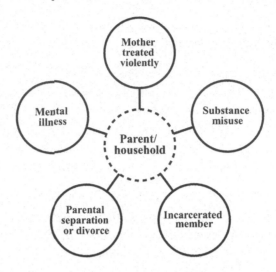

People who have been exposed to four or more ACEs are (Ashton et al, 2016):

» four times more likely to be a high-risk drinker;

» six times more likely to have had or caused unintended teenage pregnancy;

» six times more likely to smoke e-cigarettes or tobacco;

» six times more likely to have had sex under the age of 16 years;

» 11 times more likely to have smoked cannabis;

» 14 times more likely to have been a victim of violence over the past 12 months;

» 15 times more likely to have committed violence against another person in the past 12 months;

» 16 times more likely to have used crack cocaine or heroin;

» 20 times more likely to have been incarcerated at any point in their lifetime.

The ACE Pyramid (Felitti et al, 1998; CDC, 2014), shown as Figure 3.9, represents a conceptual model of the potential lifelong impact of the experience of ACEs.

Figure 3.9 ACE pyramid

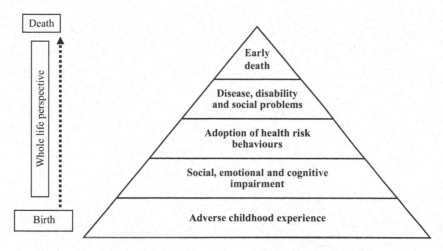

Can the effect of ACEs be moderated?

Adverse childhood experiences do not define a person; recognition of known factors is simply a tool to assist in understanding the potential risks an individual or population may face. It is possible, however, to intervene to interrupt '*the cycles of adversity*' (Bellis et al, 2014). At this point, it is important to note that while it has been evidenced that individuals who experience ACEs have an increased risk of poor outcomes as adults, as referred to above, many individuals do not go on to encounter these effects. The following factors are suggested as possible routes to the moderation of effects or impacts:

» Developing resilience through access to stable, nurturing and trusted adult–child relationships; supportive friends and being engaged in community activities, such as sports, have been shown to reduce the risk of developing mental illness, even in those people who have experienced high levels of ACEs.

» The effects of ACEs *can* last a lifetime, but they do not have to. Early identification of ACEs experienced by an individual who becomes involved with health and social care services in adulthood and supportive interventions which build trust can both reduce the impact of ACEs on the individual and also break the cycle to prevent ACEs occurring in the next generation.

» Interventions that address feelings held by the individual can be effective; examples are described in Figure 3.10.

Figure 3.10 ACE – personal thoughts and feelings

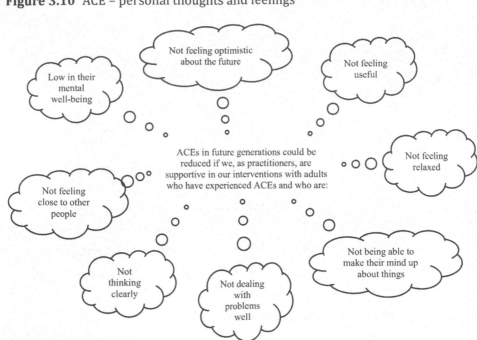

Conclusion

This chapter has been designed to give an overview of a range of issues that can, in any combination, be of particular relevance to the establishment of an empowering and respectful relationship with a person who has found themselves involved with statutory services and who may find this experience challenging and potentially threatening to their autonomy and right to self-determination. The information contained is neither definitive nor exhaustive, but more a practical summary as a 'starter for ten' for practitioners to use as a springboard to further exploration. As such, a range of resource suggestions are contained within *Taking It Further* below; we actively encourage readers to enjoy developing their own 'toolkit' of information and practice guidance for future reference in their practice.

Taking it further

References

Ainsworth, M D and Bell, S M (1970) Attachment, Exploration, and Separation: Illustrated by the Behavior of One-Year-Olds in a Strange Situation. *Journal of Child Development*, 41(1): 49–67.

Ashton, K, Bellis, M A, Davies, A R, Hardcastle, K and Hughes, K (2016) *Adverse Childhood Experiences and their Association with Chronic Disease and Health Service Use in the Welsh Adult Population*. Cardiff: Policy, Research and International Development Directorate, Public Health Wales. [online] Available at: www.wales.nhs.uk /sitesplus/documents/888/ACE%20Chronic%20Disease%20report%20%289%29%20%282%29.pdf (accessed 21 September 2020).

Bellis, M A, Hughes, K, Lackenby, N, Perkins, C and Lowey, H (2014) National Household Survey of Adverse Childhood Experiences and their Relationship with Resilience to Health-harming Behaviours in England. *BMC Medicine*, 12(1): Article 72.

Bowlby, J (1952) *Maternal Care and Mental Health*, 2nd edition. World Health Organization Monograph. [online] Available at: http://apps.who.int/iris/handle/10665/40724 (accessed 21 September 2020).

Bowlby, J (1973) *Attachment and Loss, Vol. 2: Separation*. New York, NY: Basic Books.

Bowlby, J (1982 [1969]) *Attachment and Loss, Vol. 1: Attachment*, 2nd edition. New York, NY: Basic Books.

Bretherton, I (1992) *The Origins of Attachment Theory: John Bowlby and Mary Ainsworth*. [online] Available at: www.psychology.sunysb.edu/attachment/online/inge_origins.pdf (accessed 21 September 2020).

Britten, S and Whitby, K (2018) *Self-neglect: A Practical Approach to Risks and Strengths Assessment*. St Albans: Critical Publishing.

Cassidy, J, Jones, J D and Shaver, P R (2013) Contributions of Attachment Theory and Research: A Framework for Future Research, Translation, and Policy. *Development and Psychopathology*, 25(4): 1415–34.

Centers for Disease Control and Prevention (CDC) (2014) The ACE Pyramid. Atlanta, GA: National Center for Injury Prevention and Control, Division of Violence Prevention. [online] Available at: https://web.archive.org/web/20160116162134/http://www.cdc.gov/violenceprevention/acestudy/pyramid.html (accessed 21 September 2020).

Court of Appeal (2015) *Re X (Court of Protection Practice)*. [online] Available at: www.bailii.org/ew/cases/EWCA/Civ/2015/599.html (accessed 21 September 2020).

Department for Constitutional Affairs (2005) *Mental Capacity Act 2005: Code of Practice*. London: The Stationery Office. [online] Available at: https://assets.publishing.service.gov.uk/government/uploads/system/uploads/attachment_data/file/497253/Mental-capacity-act-code-of-practice.pdf (accessed 21 September 2020).

Department for Work and Pensions and the Department of Health (2009) *Working Our Way to Better Mental Health: A Framework for Action*. London: The Stationery Office. [online] Available at: https://assets.publishing.service.gov.uk/government/uploads/system/uploads/attachment_data/file/228874/7756.pdf (accessed 21 September 2020).

Department of Health (2018) *Care and Support Statutory Guidance*. [online] Available at: www.gov.uk/government/publications/care-act-statutory-guidance/care-and-support-statutory-guidance (accessed 21 September 2020).

Felitti, V J, Anda, R F, Nordenberg, D, Williamson, D F, Spitz, A M, Edwards, V, Koss, M P and Marks, J S (1998) Relationship of Childhood Abuse and Household Dysfunction to Many of the Leading Causes of Death in Adults: The Adverse Childhood Experiences (ACE) Study. *American Journal of Preventive Medicine*, 14(4): 245–58. Available online at: www.ajpmonline.org/article/S0749-3797(98)00017-8/pdf (accessed 21 September 2020).

George, C, Kaplan, N and Main, M (1985) The Adult Attachment Interview. Unpublished manuscript. University of California at Berkeley. [online] Available at: www.psychology.sunysb.edu/attachment/measures/content/aai_interview.pdf (accessed 21 September 2020).

Heighton, A (2017) *Driving and Restraining Forces to Consider When Utilising a Conceptual Risks and Strengths Assessment Model: A Human Perspective*. Given as a presentation (unpublished).

HM Government (1983) *Mental Health Act 1983: Section 136*. Norwich: The Stationery Office. [online] Available at: www.legislation.gov.uk/ukpga/1983/20/section/136 (accessed 21 September 2020).

HM Government (1998) *Human Rights Act 1998*. Norwich: The Stationery Office. [online] Available at: www.legislation.gov.uk/ukpga/1998/42/contents (accessed 21 September 2020).

HM Government (1999) *Youth and Criminal Evidence Act 1999*. Norwich: The Stationery Office. [online] Available at: www.legislation.gov.uk/ukpga/1999/23/contents (accessed 21 September 2020).

Hughes, K, Bellis, M A, Hardcastle, K A, Sethi, D, Butchart, A, Mikton, C, Jones, L and Dunne, MP (2017) The Effect of Multiple Adverse Childhood Experiences on Health: A Systematic Review and Meta-analysis. *The Lancet Public Health*, 2(8): 356–66.

Mikulincer, M and Shaver, P (2016 [2007]) *Attachment in Adulthood: Structure, Dynamics, and Change*, 2nd edition. New York, NY: Guilford Press.

Ministry of Justice (2008) *Mental Capacity Act 2005: Deprivation of Liberty Safeguards*. London: The Stationery Office. [online] Available at: https://webarchive.nationalarchives.gov.uk/20110322122009/http://www.dh.gov.uk/en/Publicationsandstatistics/Publications/PublicationsPolicyAndGuidance/DH_085476 (accessed 21 September 2020).

National Institute for Health and Care Excellence (NICE) (2012) *Drug Use Disorders in Adults: Quality Standard (QS23)*. London and Manchester: NICE. [online] Available at: www.nice.org.uk/guidance/qs23/resources/drug-use-disorders-in-adults-pdf-2098544097733 (accessed 21 September 2020).

North Wales Safeguarding Board (NWSB) (2017) *Child Practice Reviews*. [online] Available at: www.northwalessafeguardingboard.wales/practice-reviews/child-practice-reviews/ (accessed 21 September 2020).

Perry, B and Szalavitz, M (2006) *The Boy Who Was Raised as a Dog and Other Stories from a Child Psychiatrist's Notebook: What Traumatized Children Can Teach Us About Loss, Love, and Healing*. New York, NY: Basic Books.

Rogers, C (1959) A Theory of Therapy, Personality and Interpersonal Relationships as Developed in the Client-centered Framework. In Koch, S (ed) *Psychology: A Study of a Science, Vol. 3: Formulations of the Person and the Social Context*. New York: McGraw Hill. [online] Available at: https://archive.org/stream/psychologyastudy017916mbp/psychologyastudy017916mbp_djvu.txt (accessed 21 September 2020).

Strickland, P and Allen, G (2018) *Briefing Paper Number 6337: Domestic Violence in England and Wales*. London: House of Commons. [online] Available at: https://researchbriefings.files.parliament.uk/documents/SN06337/SN06337.pdf (accessed 21 September 2020).

Supreme Court (2014) *Judgment P (by his Litigation Friend the Official Solicitor) (Appellant) v Cheshire West and Chester Council and Another (Respondents)*. [online] Available at: www.supremecourt.uk/decided-cases/docs/UKSC_2012_0068_Judgment.pdf (accessed 21 September 2020).

World Health Organization (WHO) (2018) *International Classification of Diseases – 11*. [online] Available at: www.who.int/classifications/icd/en/ (accessed 21 September 2020).

Publications

Anda, R F, Felitti, V J, Bremner, J D, Walker, J D, Whitfield, C, Perry, B D, Dube, S R and Giles, W H (2015) The Enduring Effects of Abuse and Related Adverse Experiences in Childhood: A Convergence of Evidence from Neurobiology and Epidemiology. *European Archives of Psychiatry and Clinical Neuroscience*, 256(3): 174–86.

Bowlby, J (1958) The Nature of the Child's Tie to His Mother. *International Journal of Psycho-Analysis*, 39: 350–73. [Author's notes included within the text: '*1: An abbreviated version of this paper was read before the British Psycho-Analytical Society on 19th June 1957. 2: Although in this paper I shall usually refer to mothers and not mother-figures, it is to be understood that in every case I am concerned with the person who mothers the child and to whom it becomes attached rather than to the natural mother.*']

Bowlby, J (1979) *The Making and Breaking of Affectional Bonds*. London: Tavistock Publications.

Dahmen, B, Putz, V, Herpertz-Dahlmann, B and Konrad, K (2012) Early Pathogenic Care and the Development of ADHD-like Symptoms. *Journal of Neural Transmission*, 119(9): 1023–36.

Department of Health and Social Care (2019) *Strengths-based Approach: Practice Framework and Practice Handbook*. [online] Available at: https://assets.publishing.service.gov.uk/government/uploads/system/uploads/attachment_data/file/778134/stengths-based-approach-practice-framework-and-handbook.pdf (accessed 21 September 2020).

Director of Public Prosecutions (2017) *The Code for Crown Prosecutors, Special Measures: Legal Guidance*. London: Crown Prosecution Service. [online] Available at: www.cps.gov.uk/legal-guidance/special-measures (accessed 21 September 2020).

Harding, M (2015) *Child Attachment Disorder*. Leeds: Patient Platform Ltd. [online] Available at: https://patient.info/doctor/child-attachment-disorder-pro#ref-3 (accessed 21 September 2020).

Main, M, Kaplan, N and Cassidy, J (1985) Security in Infancy, Childhood, and Adulthood: A Move to the Level of Representation. *Monographs of the Society for Research in Child Development*, 50(1/2): 66–104.

National Institute for Health and Care Excellence (NICE) (2015) *Children's Attachment: Attachment in Children and Young People Who Are Adopted from Care, in Care or at High Risk of Going into Care (NG26)*. Manchester and London: NICE. [online] Available at: www.nice.org.uk/guidance/ng26/resources/childrens-attachment-attachment-in-children-and-young-people-who-are-adopted-from-care-in-care-or-at-high-risk-of-going-into-care-pdf-1837335256261 (accessed 21 September 2020).

NHS England (2015) *Future in Mind: Promoting, Protecting and Improving Our Children's and Young People's Mental Health and Well-being*. London: Department of Health.

Obegi, J H and Berant, E (eds) (2010) *Attachment Theory and Research in Clinical Work with Adults*. New York: Guilford Press.

Reisz, S, Duschinsky, R and Siegel, D J (2018) Disorganized Attachment and Defence: Exploring John Bowlby's Unpublished Reflections. *Attachment and Human Development*, 20(2): 107–34.

Introduction

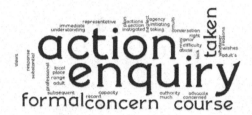

As outlined in earlier chapters, when undertaking an enquiry in safeguarding (under Section 42 of the Care Act 2014) it is necessary to establish the facts of the concern raised, if the statutory duties apply, and then in adopting an MSP approach what protective actions are required. In addition to the confirmation of an outcome to the enquiry, it is also necessary to identify if there are any ongoing concerns that there is a risk of harm or abuse occurring or of occurring in the future and if the person's desired outcome(s) have been achieved.

The Care Act (2014) and supporting *Care and Support Statutory Guidance* confirms that:

An enquiry is the action taken or instigated by the local authority in response to a concern that abuse or neglect may be taking place. An enquiry could range from a conversation with the adult, or if they lack capacity, or have substantial difficulty in understanding the enquiry their representative or advocate, prior to initiating a formal enquiry under section 42, right through to a much more formal multi-agency plan or course of action. **Whatever the course of subsequent action, the professional concerned should record the concern, the adult's views, wishes, and any immediate action has taken and the reasons for those actions.**

(Department of Health, 2018, para 14.77, emphasis added)

In this chapter, the Learning from Life case scenarios are built upon to include illustrative safeguarding adults protection plans, with an example 'Safeguarding Adults – S42 Enquiry Outcome Report' template included below (Table 4.1). This template provides a simple framework designed to enable practitioners to record the approach, and actions they have taken to establish the facts of the concern, the outcome of their enquiry and also confirmation of any further actions needed; it can be used in the absence of an agreed organisational format. The approach adopted is one based upon the strengths of the person who is alleged to have experienced or been placed at risk of experiencing harm or neglect, including consideration as applicable of their mental capacity to make their own decisions either with or without the support of an advocate. Also included is a section for the practitioner to confirm their analysis and evidence base, and how they arrived at their decision as to the conclusion of the enquiry.

Further *SnapShots on…* practitioner resources included within this chapter are:

»   The well-being principle.

»   MSP and multi-agency considerations.

SnapShot on… 'Safeguarding Adults – S42 Enquiry Outcome Report'

The Care Act requires that each local authority must:

»   *make enquiries, or cause others to do so, if it believes an adult is experiencing, or is at risk of, abuse or neglect (see para. 14.16 onwards). An enquiry should establish whether any action needs to be taken to prevent or stop abuse or neglect and if so, by who.*

(Department of Health, 2018)

Table 4.1 Example template for a 'Safeguarding Adults – S42 Enquiry Outcome Report'

Basic details	
Name of the person completing the S42 Enquiry	
Designation	
Name of agency	
Contact details	

Name of the alleged victim	
Address/location	
Gender and ethnicity	
DoB of the alleged victim	
NHS number	
Unique identification number	
Representative (Name, status/relationship, contact details)	
Date and time concern arose	
Who reported the concern? (Name, designation and contact details)	

Name of service provider (as applicable)	
Address and contact details	

Details of the Safeguarding Concern			
Include/attach body maps, medicine administration records, care plans/records, etc, as evidence			
WHAT is the concern? (confirm/cross-reference the concern report)			
WHEN did it occur? (date and time)			
WHERE did it occur? (actual location)			
WHO was involved? (names, dates of birth, gender)			
HOW did it occur? (if known)			
WHY did it occur? (if known)			
Add all additional and relevant details here:			
Mental Capacity Act (2005) and Advocacy			
1	Does the adult at risk have the Mental Capacity to decide to progress the S42 Enquiry?	YES	NO
If **YES** progress to **Question 5**			
If **NO** confirm **WHY** here, and progress to **Question 2**			
2	Has a Mental Capacity Act (2005) Assessment been completed in relation to the S42 Enquiry?	YES	NO
If **YES** attach a copy with this report and progress to **Question 3**			
If **NO** confirm **WHY** here and confirm actions to be taken and when:			
3	Has a 'Best Interests Decision' been made in relation to the progression of the S42 Enquiry?	YES	NO
If **YES** confirm **WHO** was involved and the decision made, attach a copy with this report, then progress to **Question 4**:			
If **NO** confirm **WHY** here and confirm actions to be taken and when:			
4	Does the adult at risk need the support of an advocate?	YES	NO
If **YES** confirm if this has been arranged and provided here (confirm the name and status of the advocate):			
If **NO** confirm **WHY** here:			
5	Does/will the adult at risk have 'substantial difficulty' in participating in the S42 Enquiry?	YES	NO

If **YES** confirm if advocacy has been arranged and provided here (confirm the name and status of the advocate):

Add any other relevant information here:

The adult at risk's self-expressed desired outcome(s) from the S42 Enquiry
(confirm if this was expressed with/by an advocate or representative)

What actions were taken at the time the concern was raised/known to manage the risk?
Give details of all actions that were taken to reduce/manage the risk and those to protect other adults at risk
(eg, contact with the police, health practitioners, CQC, etc)
Add additional rows as required

Date	Time	Action taken	By who	Outcome

It can be useful to start a 'Chronology of Events Log' to give a clear overall picture of events

(start at the earliest date and work forwards)

Chronology of Events Log

Date and time	Source of evidence	Event	People involved	Actions/ decisions taken	Significance

Add additional rows as required

The S42 Enquiry Action Plan

Give details of what you plan to do to complete the S42 Enquiry, including people you plan to interview.

Enquiry Action Plan Template:

Date	Time	Action	By who	Outcome

Add additional rows as required

Analysis and decision-making

Describe the analysis you have undertaken following the collation of all applicable information and HOW you have arrived at your decision.

Confirmation that the adult at risk's desired outcomes have been achieved

The outcome of the S42 Enquiry	
Confirm all actions taken and those planned as a result. This may include disciplinary action with a member of staff; referral to a professional regulatory body (eg, Nursing and Midwifery Council (NMC) or the Disclosure and Barring Service (DBS)); additional training or supervision; updating Care Plans and/or Risk Assessment; review of prescribed medicines; etc.	

The outcome of the S42 Enquiry	
Actions required	
Actions taken	

Add additional rows as required

Any Next Steps?
Include any lessons learned; this may be changes in policy, procedures, training plans, etc, actions you plan to take and importantly how you will monitor improvements.

Next Steps – Action Plan and Monitoring Arrangements Template:

Date	Action	By who?	When?	Outcome confirmed

Add additional rows as required

Date S42 Enquiry Outcome Report completed	
Signature	

The contents of this document are confidential; compliance with all applicable legislation and the General Data Protection Regulations (Information Commissioner's Office, 2018) must be maintained at all times.

Principles in care and support planning and protection plans

Where it is found that there is a need for further work to be undertaken, and in order to plan effective and proportionate protection with the person for the future, the core principles of person-centred and person-led care and support planning should be followed as an empowering and enabling approach.

The following practice pointers can assist in forming the basis for the design of all Care and Support Plans, and can act as a set of principles to inform the person-centred and person-led development and agreement of a safeguarding adults protection plan.

» Always start with the adult and their rights at the forefront.

» The adult's mental capacity has been assessed in line with the requirements of the Mental Capacity Act (2005); this is clearly documented with best interests decision-making as applicable.

» Confirm that all decisions made regarding the adult's mental capacity and their need, or not, for the support of an advocate are fully documented – this includes circumstances where the adult may experience significant difficulty in being fully involved.

» A proportionate assessment of the adult's needs has been completed in line with the Care Act (2014) duties, with an indicative personal budget amount outlined.

» The 'well-being principle' and the adult's voice is evidenced throughout the Care and Support Plan.

» The protected characteristics of the adult have been recognised and respected, with necessary adjustments made as/when required.

» Innovative and creative thinking has been employed – this evidences consideration and action taken to make arrangements that will best support the adult to be fully involved and direct how their needs can be met.

» The Care and Support Plan details, in the adult's own words, how they wish to stay well, healthy and safe by confirming their goals and outcomes and how they will be achieved.

» Informal carers have contributed to care and support planning as applicable; they have been offered an assessment (either jointly with the adult or individually) of their needs in sustaining their role, with contingency planning should their contribution become unavailable for whatever reason.

» If a carer is involved with the adult, support and encourage them to have an assessment of their own needs – sometimes carers don't recognise how vital their role is and can be concerned that an assessment is a test of their abilities.

» Contingency planning and 'what if ...' conversations can, at times, be difficult to initiate, but if undertaken positively can prove immensely useful in avoiding crisis situations and act as a real reassurance to the adult and their carer. This can be a key priority for an adult who experiences fluctuations in their mental capacity, eg: *'When I lack the mental capacity to make decisions for myself, this is how I want to be supported, and by who...'* Consider the use of a 'Choice and Control' Advance Care and Support Plan (Britten and Whitby, 2018).

» A strengths-based risk assessment approach in care and support planning that explores all natural assets and resources available to the adult to meet their needs and desired outcomes should be taken – this may include the use of assistive technologies, local community or personal assets/resources, signposting or the provision of other information resources.

» The adult has been given the opportunity to design their own Care and Support Plan in their chosen format.

» The Care and Support Plan details how eligible needs will be met within the indicative personal budget initially calculated as part of the Care Act Assessment process; the finalised personal budget should be confirmed at the end of the care and support planning process and give a clear breakdown of how costings have been calculated and which care/support element they refer to.

» As applicable, non-eligible needs and personal aspirations should also be included, with confirmation of how they will be met.

» The adult and/or their representative must receive a copy of their Care and Support Plan; as applicable it confirms who, when and how it will be reviewed.

What *good* looks like in care and support planning

The *Care and Support Statutory Guidance* (Department of Health, 2018) includes a link to an initiative undertaken by Think Local Act Personal (2014) called *Delivering Care and Support Planning*. This online publication is part of a suite of resources commissioned by the Department of Health in partnership with the Local Government Association and the Association of Directors of Adult Social Services to the implementation of the Care Act (2014).

Included within *Delivering Care and Support Planning* are ten statements of principle entitled 'What good looks like in care and support planning' (Figure 4.1); these were developed in co-production with people with care and support needs, carers and family members, and they very much echo and support the 'practice pointers' above.

Figure 4.1 Think Local Act Personal (2014): what good looks like in care and support planning

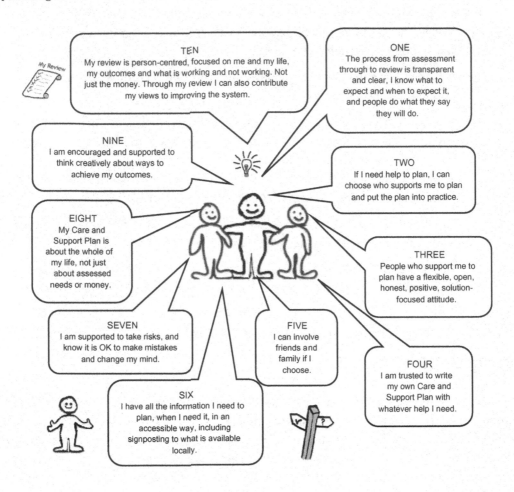

Learning from Life case scenarios

Scenario one – JA

The initial information-gathering and subsequent enquiry into the Safeguarding Concern submitted by the Environmental Health department were found to be true – JA was living in a home environment which was insanitary and extremely cluttered; this was a case of self-neglect. The risk levels identified following the collation of all relevant information were confirmed as follows:

Mental health	Critical/immediate level of risk
Physical health	Critical/immediate level of risk
Environment and housing	Critical/immediate level of risk
Social network	Moderate level of risk
Exploitation/abuse	High level of risk
Early life experiences	Low level of risk

JA maintained his involvement and became motivated to confirm supportive and protective arrangements. JA had been confirmed as eligible for and in need of care and support; immediate action was taken to confirm a personal budget to meet his desired outcomes. A protection plan was created by JA, with his advocate, as his clear account of how it was agreed he would be supported. An example format is given in Table 4.2.

Table 4.2 Safeguarding adults protection plan – JA

Details of person completing plan	Safeguarding adults protection plan		
Name: **			
Contact details: ******			
	Person to be supported		
Name: 'Learning from Life' JA			**Gender:** Male
Current address: ***	**Post code:** ***		
	Telephone number: ***		
Relevant ID number: ***	**Date of implementation of plan:** **/**/****		
Outcome desired	**Action needed**	**Person responsible**	**Timescale**
In response to a Safeguarding Concern submitted **/**/**** *I want to be able to live safely and independently in my own home, with recognition of the individual type of support I need in relation to my known diagnoses.*	JA to be supported to maintain clarity about how his personal budget can be spent.	Social worker JA JA's advocate	Ongoing to next review
	JA to be supported to recruit a team of staff (within his personal budget) who have training and experience of 'Autism spectrum disorder without disorder of intellectual development and with mild or no impairment of functional language'.	JA JA's advocate	Immediate
	JA to be supported to create and maintain a pictorial calendar of planned activities.	JA JA's family All staff supporting JA	Ongoing to next review

JA to be supported to fulfil his responsibilities as a tenant by maintaining his home environment (internal and external) and to reduce the opportunity for exploitation, doorstep scamming and mate/hate crime.	JA JA's support staff	Immediate and ongoing to next review
JA to be supported to access and attend primary and secondary health services as planned; this also includes dentist, optician, etc.	JA JA's support staff	Ongoing to next review
JA to receive advice and support from **** Fire and Rescue Service about fire safety in the home.	JA JA's advocate	Immediate
JA to be supported to plan, purchase and prepare a nutritionally balanced diet.	JA JA's support staff	Ongoing to next review
JA to be supported to create and maintain an accurate list of people to contact when he experiences difficulties.	JA JA's advocate	Immediate and ongoing to next review
All visits to JA to be arranged with him in advance – all new people to send a photograph to him before they visit.	All people supporting JA	Immediate and ongoing to next review
All people involved to be aware that before sending any information in relation to the planning or delivery of support via the postal service they must telephone JA in advance to let him know – receiving unexpected written information of this type is detrimental to his mental health and well-being	All people supporting JA	Immediate and ongoing to next review
JA to be supported to mitigate the risks of social isolation by supporting him to engage in his range of interests and hobbies.	JA JA's support staff	Ongoing to next review

Preventative strategies	Regular pre-booked visits/telephone contact by: • social worker • advocate • nominated professionals And responses to: • contact initiated by JA
Indications/triggers for further concern	**Triggers** to a decline in JA's mental health and well-being are varied; however, they include any activities outside of the usual boundaries and plans JA has set for himself. JA's level of distress can also vary because of his sensitivities to particular sounds, at particular times – JA will initially alert people about the impact particular sounds are having on him. When JA is experiencing a decline in his mental health and well-being he will react by excessive head-banging, slapping himself, swearing and screaming unpredictably; he will also telephone his mother and any people involved with him to inform them that he intends to kill himself – this can be at any time throughout the day or at night.
Contingency plan	In the event of the indicators above occurring the *** Crisis Team must be contacted and welfare **telephone contact** made with JA to determine whether an assessment under the Mental Health Act (1983) is required. An increase in contact with JA should be negotiated – this contact to be either pre-booked telephone or face to face visits.
Review date:	**/**/****

Please retain one copy on person's file and forward a copy to: ****

Completed by:	JA		Date completed: **/**/****
	Advocate Social worker		

Scenario two – CD

The enquiry into the Safeguarding Concern, undertaken under Section 42 of the Care Act (2014), concluded that the allegation of financial exploitation/abuse was inconclusive; however, in discussing the issues with CD, she felt that she wanted further support to enable her to develop personal safety strategies for the future. CD felt that she had not been able to involve herself positively within her local community and would like her existing Care and Support Plan to be reviewed in light of her recent experiences, and the re-emergence of feelings of low self-worth, isolation and loneliness which she felt led her into situations where she misinterpreted and misjudged the motivations of others; this she linked with her early life experiences.

Mental health	Critical/immediate level of risk
Physical health	High level of risk
Environment and housing	High level of risk
Social network	Moderate level of risk
Exploitation/abuse	Critical/immediate level of risk
Early life experiences	Critical/immediate level of risk

The actions identified by and confirmed with CD to be undertaken are confirmed in Table 4.3.

Table 4.3 Safeguarding adults protection plan – CD

Details of person completing plan	Safeguarding adults protection plan
Name: **	
Contact details: ******	
	Person to be supported
Name: 'Learning from Life' CD	**Date of birth:** **/**/**** **Gender:** Female
Current address: ***	**Post code:** ***
	Telephone number: ***
Relevant ID number: ***	**Date of implementation of plan:** **/**/****

Outcome desired	Action needed	Person responsible	Timescale
In response to a Safeguarding Concern submitted **/**/**** *I would like to be supported to develop my own life-skills and awareness to keep myself safe in the future and to build my confidence to live independently.*	CD to be supported to access the local 'Mindfulness and Emotional Coping Skills' programme run by the community mental health trust.	Social worker CD Support worker	Initial six-session programme to start on **/**/****
	CD to be supported to explore and identify opportunities for volunteering and skill development with the local Dogs Trust.	CD Support worker	Immediate and ongoing to next review
	Review of existing Care and Support Plan to reflect CD's strengths and required outcomes identified as part of the S42 Enquiry.	CD Advocate Social worker	By the next review date
	Home Safety Check to be arranged with the local Fire and Rescue Service.	Social worker CD Support worker	Immediate and ongoing to next review
	CD to attend the next 'Neighbourhood Watch' meeting and decide if this will assist her in getting to know her neighbours better and to build her confidence in the community.	CD Support worker	**/**/**

Preventative strategies	CD to maintain contact with her advocate and raise any concerns or queries she has with her support worker and/or social worker as applicable.
Indications/triggers for further concern	CD described that when she initially experiences a decline in her mental health and sense of well-being, she will isolate herself and become demotivated and withdrawn; if the decline continues, she is then drawn back to a pattern of self-harming behaviours. CD needs her support workers to remain vigilant for these signs.
Contingency plan	In the event that the indicators above occur the social worker and community health should be contacted.
Review date:	****/**/**** (six weeks from the date of this plan)**

Please retain one copy on person's file and forward a copy to: ****

Completed by:		Date completed:	**/**/****
CD			
	Advocate		
	Social Worker		

Practice matters

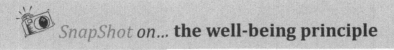

SnapShot on... **the well-being principle**

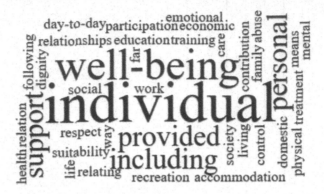

This *SnapShot* is designed to give practitioners an overview of the Care Act (2014) requirements as an aid to the further development and enhancement of person-centred and person-focused practice.

The key factors of 'well-being' specified within the Care Act (2014) and supporting statutory guidance, to be considered throughout all interventions, are shown in Figure 4.2 – there is no hierarchy of elements, and all should be considered as applicable to the individual person with whom a care and support plan is being undertaken.

The *Care and Support Statutory Guidance* contains the following directions:

1.2 *Local authorities **must promote wellbeing** when carrying out any of their care and support functions in respect of a person. This may sometimes be referred to as 'the wellbeing principle' because it is a guiding principle that puts wellbeing at the heart of care and support.*

1.3 *The wellbeing principle **applies in all cases** where a local authority is carrying out a care and support function or making a decision, in relation to a person. For this reason, it is referred to throughout this guidance. It applies equally to adults with care and support needs **and their carers**.*

(Department of Health, 2018, paras 1.2 - 1.3)

Figure 4.2 The well-being principle wheel

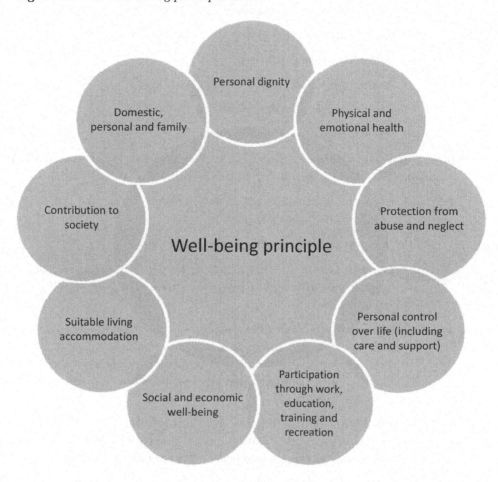

The Care Act (2014) Part 1 'General responsibilities of local authorities' details all of the elements which must be promoted when undertaking social care interventions.

Promoting individual well-being

(1)   *The general duty of a local authority, in exercising a function under this Part in the case of an individual, is to promote that individual's well-being.*

(2)   *'Well-being', in relation to an individual, means that individual's well-being so far as relating to any of the following –*

    (a)   personal dignity (including treatment of the individual with respect);

    (b)   physical and mental health and emotional well-being;

    (c)   protection from abuse and neglect;

(d)   *control by the individual over day-to-day life (including over care and support, or support, provided to the individual and the way in which it is provided);*

(e)   *participation in work, education, training or recreation;*

(f)   *social and economic well-being;*

(g)   *domestic, family and personal relationships;*

(h)   *suitability of living accommodation;*

(i)   *the individual's contribution to society.*

(3)   *In exercising a function under this Part in the case of an individual, a local authority must have regard to the following matters in particular –*

(a)   *the importance of beginning with the assumption that the individual is best-placed to judge the individual's well being;*

(b)   *the individual's views, wishes, feelings and beliefs;*

(c)   *the importance of preventing or delaying the development of needs for care and support or needs for support and the importance of reducing needs of either kind that already exist;*

(d)   *the need to ensure that decisions about the individual are made having regard to all the individual's circumstances (and are not based only on the individual's age or appearance or any condition of the individual's or aspect of the individual's behaviour which might lead others to make unjustified assumptions about the individual's well-being);*

(e)   *the importance of the individual participating as fully as possible in decisions relating to the exercise of the function concerned and being provided with the information and support necessary to enable the individual to participate;*

(f)   *the importance of achieving a balance between the individual's well-being and that of any friends or relatives who are involved in caring for the individual;*

(g)   *the need to protect people from abuse and neglect;*

(h)   *the need to ensure that any restriction on the individual's rights or freedom of action that is involved in the exercise of the function is kept to the minimum necessary for achieving the purpose for which the function is being exercised.*

(HM Government, 2014, Part 1 Section 1)

These statutory duties require little, if any explanation; however, it may be useful to include here the translation to person-centred practice pointers for use by practitioners:

» Building on the principles of the Mental Capacity Act (2005), the local authority should assume that the person themself knows best their own outcomes, goals and well-being. Local authorities should not make assumptions as to what matters most to the person.

» Considering the person's views and wishes is critical to a person-centred system. Local authorities should not ignore or downplay the importance of a person's own opinions in relation to their life and their care. Where particular views, feelings or beliefs (including religious beliefs) impact on the choices that a person may wish to make about their care, these should be taken into account. This is especially important where a person has expressed views in the past, but no longer has the capacity to make decisions themselves.

» At every interaction with a person, a local authority should consider whether or how the person's needs could be reduced, or other needs could be delayed from arising. Effective interventions at the right time can stop needs from escalating, and help people maintain their independence for longer.

» Local authorities should not make judgements based on preconceptions about the person's circumstances (based only on their age or appearance, any condition they have or any aspect of their behaviour that might lead others to make unjustified assumptions about their well-being) but should in every case work to understand their individual needs and goals.

» The information and support necessary should be provided to enable the individual to participate in decisions about them. Care and support should be personal, and local authorities should not make decisions from which the person is excluded.

» People should be considered in the context of their families and support networks, not just as isolated individuals with needs. Local authorities should take into account the impact of an individual's need on those who support them and take steps to help others access information or support.

» In any activity that a local authority undertakes, it should consider how to ensure that the person is and remains protected from abuse or neglect. This is not confined only to safeguarding issues but should be a general principle applied in every case, including with those who self-neglect.

» Where the local authority has to take actions which restrict rights or freedoms, they should ensure that the course followed is the least restrictive necessary. Concerns about self-neglect do not override this principle.

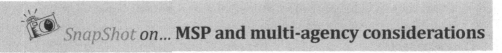

SnapShot on... **MSP and multi-agency considerations**

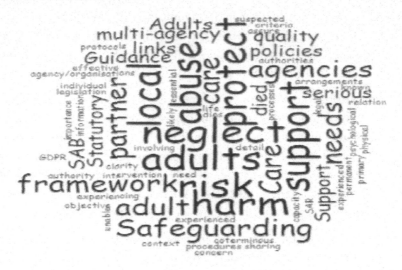

This *SnapShot* aims to support and expand practitioners' thinking in their exploration of the dynamics of working within the multi-agency context of safeguarding adults. It considers the positive benefits of collaborative approaches to what are and can be the challenges that arise due to, in some part, for example, differences in terminology, understanding, perspectives and perceptions of roles and responsibilities.

What is multi-agency working?

Multi-agency working is where an agency combines their skills, knowledge and expertise with one or more others, around the common aim of meeting an individual's needs – this is also applicable to situations that relate to the needs of a group of people who are at risk of harm or neglect, for example in a supported living or residential care setting. In this particular context, we are referring to safeguarding goals and risk management strategies.

Why is it important?

Timely and effective multi-agency working underpins a positive approach to information-sharing and decision-making within the safeguarding arena. This, in turn, can prove immensely effective in mitigating against and preventing abuse as well as in identifying patterns and/or prevalence of sources of harm.

The new statutory framework clarifies and enhances the duties, roles and responsibilities of local authorities and their partners. It strengthens the multi-agency strategic and collaborative approach to adult safeguarding and is not simply a continuation of business as usual.

(Crawley, 2015, p 151)

The *Care and Support Statutory Guidance* gives clear direction regarding statutory expectations and duties for '*integration, cooperation and partnerships*' placed upon local authorities in England.

Co-operation of partner organisations

Paragraph 15.15

All public organisations should work together and co-operate where needed, in order to ensure a focus on the care and support (including carers' support) and health and health-related needs of their local population. Whilst there are some local services where the local authority must actively promote integration, in other cases it must nonetheless co-operate with relevant local and national partners.

Paragraph 15.16

Co-operation between partners should be a general principle for all those concerned, and all should understand the reasons why co-operation is important for those people involved. The Act sets out 5 aims of co-operation between partners which are relevant to care and support, although it should be noted that the purposes of co-operation are not limited to these matters:

» *promoting the well-being of adults needing care and support and of carers*

» *improving the quality of care and support for adults and support for carers (including the outcomes from such provision)*

» *smoothing the transition from children's to adults' services*

» *protecting adults with care and support needs who are currently experiencing or at risk of abuse or neglect*

» *identifying lessons to be learned from cases where adults with needs for care and support have experienced serious abuse or neglect.*

(Department of Health, 2018, para 15.15)

The authors advocate the promotion of the following principles as essential features in safeguarding the welfare and well-being of adults at risk.

» To embed a shared understanding of the tasks, processes and roles outlined in both statutory and local requirements for the safeguarding of adults at risk.

» To create effectively integrated working arrangements at strategic and individual operational levels across services.

» To agree safe and effective communication channels and mechanisms across agencies, which include a commitment to common key definitions, terminology and thresholds for intervention.

» To ensure sound decision-making based on effective information-sharing, a thorough assessment of need, risk analysis and professional judgement.

Consideration of the positives and negatives of multi-agency working

The advantages of effective multi-agency working can include:

» timely and accurate information-sharing;

» early identification of issues or concerns which may require intervention;

» streamlined and obstacle-free access to services, skills, knowledge and subject matter expertise;

» shared ownership of decision-making and responsibility;

» the co-ordination of responses that incorporate and reflect different agencies' perspectives.

The disadvantages of multi-agency working can include:

» a lack of commitment from agencies;

» an absence of clarity in relation to respective roles and responsibilities which can result in disagreements and conflict;

» untimely, ineffective and inaccurate information-sharing;

» a lack of consistency of intervention, which negatively impacts on the delivery of care/support.

Safeguarding Adults Boards in England

The Care Act (2014) and accompanying *Care and Support Statutory Guidance* (Department of Health, 2018) set out the legal framework that surrounds how agencies are required to work to protect adults at risk of abuse or neglect. This legislation placed Safeguarding Adults Boards (SABs) on a statutory footing, with the requirement that local authorities set up a SAB in their area.

A primary objective of the SAB is to assure itself that local safeguarding arrangements and partner agencies act to support and protect adults in their area who:

» have needs for care and support (whether or not the local authority is meeting any of those needs); *and*

» are experiencing or at risk of abuse or neglect; *and*

» as a result of their need for care and support are unable to protect themselves from either the risk or experience of abuse or neglect.

High-quality multi-agency working is essential to the effective implementation of the statutory safeguarding adults framework. Each local Safeguarding Adults Board (SAB) should detail, within their policies and procedures, how their framework for multi-agency working – in responding to concerns regarding adults at risk of abuse, harm or neglect – links to and is coterminous with each partner agency/organisation's own internal processes and policies. These links and clarity are of particular importance in relation to information-sharing protocols and the General Data Protection Regulations (Information Commissioner's Office, 2018).

When the requirements and criteria for a Safeguarding Adults Review (SAR) are met, the local SAB has responsibility for commissioning a review. The aim of the SAR is to understand what happened, to learn lessons and to identify and implement ways of improving working practice in single and/or multi-agency settings. The SAR criteria are contained within Chapter 14 of the *Care and Support Statutory Guidance*:

Paragraph 14.162

SABs must arrange a SAR when an adult in its area dies as a result of abuse or neglect, whether known or suspected, and there is concern that partner agencies could have worked more effectively to protect the adult.

Paragraph 14.163

SABs must also arrange a SAR if an adult in its area has not died, but the SAB knows or suspects that the adult has experienced serious abuse or neglect. In the context of SARs, something can be considered serious abuse or neglect where, for example the individual would have been likely to have died but for an intervention, or has suffered permanent harm or has reduced capacity or quality of life (whether because of physical or psychological effects) as a result of the abuse or neglect. SABs are free to arrange for a SAR in any other situations involving an adult in its area with needs for care and support.

(Department of Health, 2018)

Taking it further

References

Crawley, C (2015) A View from the Department of Health. *Journal of Adult Protection*, 17(3): 151–2.

Department of Health (2018) *Care and Support Statutory Guidance*. [online] Available at: www.gov.uk/government/publications/care-act-statutory-guidance/care-and-support-statutory-guidance (accessed 21 September 2020).

HM Government (2014) *The Care Act 2014*. Norwich: The Stationery Office. [online] Available at: www.legislation.gov.uk/ukpga/2014/23/pdfs/ukpga_20140023_en.pdf (accessed 21 September 2020).

Information Commissioner's Office (2018) *Guide to the General Data Protection Regulations*. [online] Available at: www.gov.uk/government/publications/guide-to-the-general-data-protection-regulation (accessed 21 September 2020).

Think Local Act Personal (2014) *Delivering Care and Support Planning*. [online] Available at: www.thinklocalactpersonal.org.uk/_assets/Resources/SDS/TLAPCareSupportPlanning.pdf (accessed 21 September 2020).

Publications

Association of Directors of Adult Social Services (ADASS) (2005) *Safeguarding Adults: A National Framework for Good Practice and Outcomes in Adult Protection.* [online] Available at: www.adass.org.uk/AdassMedia/stories/Publications/Guidance/safeguarding.pdf (accessed 21 September 2020).

Association of Directors of Adult Social Services (ADASS) (2018) *Making Safeguarding Personal Outcomes Framework: Final Report.* [online] Available at: www.adass.org.uk/media/6525/msp-outcomes-framework-final-report-may-2018.pdf (accessed 21 September 2020).

Atkinson, A, Jones, M and Lamont, E (2007) *Multi-agency Working and its Implications for Practice: A Review of the Literature.* Reading: CfBT Education Trust. [online] Available at: www.nfer.ac.uk/publications/MAD01/MAD01.pdf (accessed 21 September 2020).

Preston-Shoot, M (2015) *Safeguarding in Light of the Care Act.* Totnes: Research in Practice for Adults (RiPfA).

Websites

Research in Practice: www.ripfa.org.uk/resources/training-and-events/commissioned-workshops/menu-workshops/menu-workshop-outcomes-approach-into-practice/ (accessed 21 September 2020).

Introduction

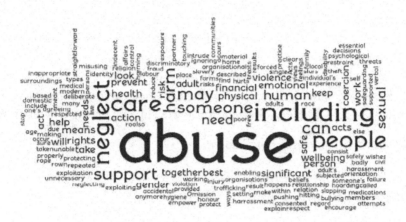

The management of known risk is a complex matter in all aspects of practice, particularly in situations where, as an outcome of a Safeguarding Adults Enquiry or as part of care and support assessment or planning, there is the identified risk of extremely serious injury or death of an adult at risk who holds the mental capacity to make their own decisions, and they refuse to engage with the planning and delivery of vital care and support.

It is worth here to restate the statutory safeguarding duties, taken directly from the *Care and Support Statutory Guidance* (Department of Health, 2018, para 14.2):

The safeguarding duties apply to an adult who:

»   *Has needs for care and support (whether or not the local authority is meeting any of those needs)*

»   *Is experiencing, or at risk of, abuse or neglect*

»   *As a result of those care and support needs is unable to protect themselves from either the risk of, or the experience of abuse or neglect*

This chapter considers aspects of risk management with those adults who meet the criteria specified above, and who:

>   »   hold the mental capacity to make their own decisions;

>   »   have made, and continue to make, decisions that place them at risk of extremely serious injury or death;

>   »   refuse to engage with vital care and support services.

It is explicit here that all aspects of and approaches to person-centred practice will have been exhausted. In these circumstances, the human rights of the adult at risk must be respected by all practitioners involved; however, practitioners (and the agencies/organisations they work for) must also ensure that they have explored all available avenues to appropriately and proportionately safeguard the person and promote their well-being, independence and autonomy.

Many local authorities and Safeguarding Adults Boards (SABs) will have developed their own approaches to this complex area of practice, and where operational arrangements and procedures do exist these should be followed by practitioners. Our aim here is to highlight some key practice topics for consideration, which include an overview of basic human responses that adults may make when faced with interventions in their life and the legal principle of inherent jurisdiction, and to give a simple flowchart depiction of when and how to initiate what we refer to as a 'Multi-agency Risk Management Meeting' in order to discuss, confirm and document a clear, effective and proportionate plan to address the risk identified.

The *SnapShots on...* contained in this chapter are:

> » Risk aversion.

> » Information-sharing.

> » Dispute resolution.

> » The coroner and reports under Regulation 28.

Driving and restraining forces to consider when utilising a conceptual risks and strengths assessment model: a human perspective

Consultant psychiatrist Dr Andrew Heighton (MBChB, MRCPsych), in a presentation he gave in September 2017, described that any intervention to support a person who has experienced or is at risk of harm or neglect will inevitably be challenging for all practitioners, particularly when they refuse that support. The intervention may well be perceived as a 'threat' to the person concerned, as well as it being an opportunity for potential personal growth and life-enhancing change. As humans we have a tendency to focus more acutely on 'threats' to our personal survival; this predisposition may pose significant challenges for any professional involved in supporting a person who is being, or is at risk of, abuse or neglect (including self-neglect).

Evolutionary perspective

Humans have evolved to be very sensitive to a perceived threat in their own environment; the 'survival instinct':

- » flight;
- » fight;
- » freeze.

In general, a situation which is perceived to be 'too different' can, for some, equate to a 'threat to their survival'. It is therefore essential to ensure that any intervention considers and incorporates this factor. Being faced with 'too much difference' can trigger a person's 'survival instinct' to keep themselves and their environment, in their terms, safe and stable. This response, in turn, can reduce the person's capacity to process and manage new information and experiences; this may also create resistance to any suggestion of change.

Roles and goals

Each and every intervention should be based upon clear and specific goals, in order to establish a context. These can be expressed as:

- » **explicit goals:** for example, to create a safe sleeping environment within a home that is extremely cluttered;
- » **implicit goals:** for example, to survive, to keep the situation stable, versus to grow and develop.

If the *explicit* goal to be achieved is not clearly specified and understood, there is an increased risk of triggering the *implicit* goal to survive, and thus progress will be impeded and create challenges for both the person at the centre of the intervention and the person supporting.

As humans we need meaning; the following simple questions to ask ourselves are useful in establishing reasons for change.

- » *What* is the reason for doing things this way?
- » *Why* do things need to change?

If roles are not clear, *how* does the person at the centre of the intervention know what they need to do? They may believe that someone else is responsible for the action; this in itself may meet their personal implicit goal to convince themselves that the required action is someone else's job/responsibility.

Survive *or* thrive?

The ability to keep a person receptive to new experiences is a vital component of the successful navigation of positive change and achieving 'the best' out of a situation that a person may not necessarily want to fully embrace.

The person at the centre of the intervention may react against the authority held by the person responsible for the instigation of necessary change. Resistance to change can be triggered by many and varying factors, for example:

- » an instruction or request;
- » tone of voice, word choice, 'a saying';
- » facial expression, a gesture;
- » sensory experiences such as smells or noises.

The person may react in compliance or act defiantly; both of these are survival responses and are likely to come from a place where the person is less able to learn and develop from the process. These are both normal human reactions – don't take it personally.

Impact?

The complexity of managing human interactions, especially in situations where a person has mental capacity and is, for example, severely self-neglecting, can open up gaps in information-sharing. This in itself can potentially lead to increased risk such as:

- » delays in decision-making;
- » factors/information missed;
- » people being invalidated;
- » complaints and further Safeguarding Concerns being raised;
- » it is a virtual 'minefield';
- » technical solutions rarely solve non-technical problems;
- » it is difficult to devise an action or protection plan that encompasses values and feelings.

In considering the factors described by Dr Heighton (2017), to actualise the principles of MSP, practitioners may wish to develop their own awareness further. The relevance and use of approaches such as 'motivational interviewing' may be worth exploring.

Topics for consideration and exploration

Inherent jurisdiction

Practitioners who are working with adults who have the mental capacity to make specific decisions at the time they need to be made, which result in them placing themselves at risk of serious and significant harm or death may, occasionally, be required to consider the use of intervention by the law courts to protect the safety of that person. In situations such as this while giving careful consideration of person-centredness and proportionality, the legal principle of 'inherent jurisdiction' may arise and be of relevance; practitioners should always seek and secure the formal legal opinion, advice and input of an appropriately qualified and experienced legal professional.

In brief, inherent jurisdiction is a principle/rule of common law in England that the High Court (or more superior court, such as the Court of Appeal, or higher) has the right and power to hear cases and make legal judgments on any matter that is not held under the jurisdiction of another court or tribunal.

The common law is the great safety net which lies behind all statute law and is capable of filling gaps left by that law, if and in so far as those gaps have to be filled in the interests of society as a whole. This process of using the common law to fill gaps is one of the most important duties of the judges.

(House of Lords, 1990, np)

In order to give this description practical meaning in the context of safeguarding and mental capacity, it will be useful for practitioners to read in full the judgment given by Lord Justice Baker in the Court of Appeal on 21 December 2018, regarding a case brought by a local authority and a 97 year-old man referred to as BF. This case also includes consideration of the interplay and interrelationship of 'inherent jurisdiction' and Article 5 of the Human Rights Act (1998). The link to the full judgment in this case (Court of Appeal, 2018) is contained within the *Taking It Further* section at the end of this chapter; however, a summary of this scenario is given below as an aid to building context of this highly complex legal issue. It must be noted that this is a brief summary that does not contain all details of the case heard by the High Court or the Court of Appeal, and is not based upon qualified legal interpretation, more it is to provide practice insight. As emphasised above, formal legal advice and input should always be sought on a case by case basis.

Summary:

> » BF was a 97 year-old man who had various physical health conditions including blindness; he had the mental capacity to decide where and how he lived. For many years, following the death of his wife, he lived with his son KF. KF was known to have serious alcohol and drug addictions, and his behaviours placed his father at serious risk of harm or even, it was recognised, death. These behaviours were both abusive and neglectful, in that he and BF lived in insanitary conditions. The

local authority started legal proceedings in the High Court, under inherent jurisdiction in March 2017.

» BF was eligible for care and support from the local authority, and a Care and
Support Plan was in place to provide him with support with essential personal
hygiene needs and to support his dietary intake. However, as a consequence of
KF's behaviours and also the reported lack of co-operation of BF, care providers
were unable to continue to provide their services, even though extensive efforts
were made to put in place and sustain alternative arrangements over a consider-
able period of time.

» In May 2018, the local authority made applications to the High Court, under
'*inherent jurisdiction*' for '*a declaration that having done all that could be reason-
ably done to provide BF with care, it should be discharged from all duties owed
to him*'. Their application was granted. It was confirmed that the local authority
would continue to be responsible for the delivery of a meal to BF each day, and
that should he change his mind, BF would make contact with them.

» Within a few months (September 2018), BF experienced severe deterioration in
his health and home environment – he was persuaded to move to a care home
for a period of respite care. At this time, the local authority was concerned that
BF may have lost his capacity to make decisions about where he lived; they made
a further application to the High Court and an order was granted that restrained
BF from returning to his own home or living with his son, KF, and required him to
remain living at the care home until further notice.

» BF was confirmed to hold the mental capacity to decide his own living arrangements and in December 2018, the local authority sought a lifting of the injunc-
tions imposed by the High Court on BF; this was refused.

» Matters relating to a potential infringement of BF's rights under Article 5 (right
to liberty and security) of the Human Rights Act (1998) were raised, in that the
case fell outside of the scope of inherent jurisdiction; however, Lord Justice Baker,
when hearing the case in the Court of Appeal (a superior court to the High Court),
concluded that the decision made by the High Court to refuse the lifting of the
injunction was not wrong.

Multi-agency risk management process

In the context of work with adults with care and support needs who are eligible for support
from the local authority and whose refusal to engage with care and support planning or the
delivery of essential support services places them at serious risk of life-threatening abuse or
neglect (including self-neglect), it is probable that other agencies may also be involved; for
example healthcare, housing agencies or potentially the police.

Figure 5.1 Example multi-agency risk management/decision-making framework

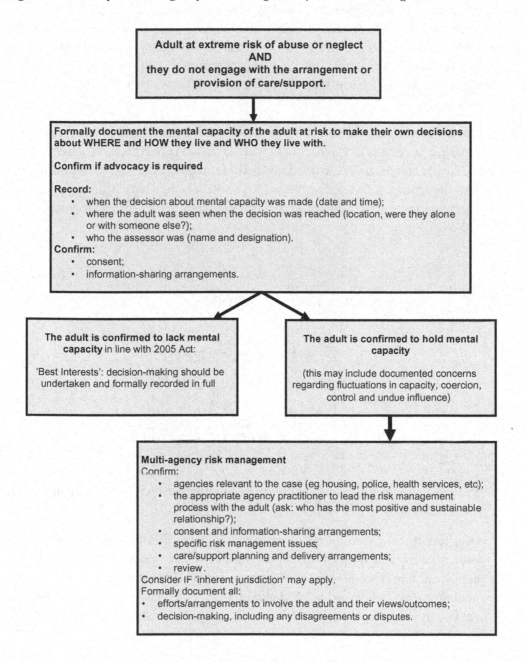

The adoption of a person-centred and strengths-based approach to all interventions, as expanded upon in earlier chapters of this text, places vital importance upon consideration and evaluation of the potential source or causes for their refusal. When all efforts and options to enable and empower the person to be involved in managing their own safety strategies have been exhausted it may, at times, be necessary to convene a multi-agency risk management planning meeting including and involving wherever and however possible the person themself. The adoption of a multi-agency response in these types of circumstances supports a broader view to be gained of the wider implications and resources applicable to the individual case. This can be of great relevance in situations where coercive control may be a factor of exploitation, abuse or neglect where the police could be of direct assistance.

A basis for decision-making and planning to initiate a multi-agency risk management planning meeting is suggested in Figure 5.1. As with all planning processes, required actions should be clearly and concisely recorded, giving confirmation of the person responsible for completing the action, the timescale within which it will be completed and arrangements for reviewing the outcome of the actions taken (What, Why, How, Who, When and, as applicable, Where).

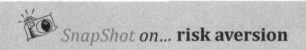

SnapShot on... **risk aversion**

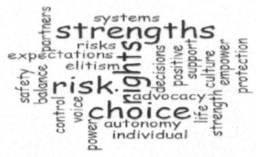

The most effective organisations are those adopting positive, rather than defensive, approaches to risk.

Over recent years, with the development of the personalisation agenda and heightened awareness of safeguarding adults' duties, we have, as professionals in health and social care, become increasingly preoccupied with risk. There is a view that minimising risk, and even the avoidance of 'risky' decisions, is the safest strategy to employ in order to protect an adult at risk – at times, for some, the concept of risk equates to harm.

The graphic representations below outline some of the concerns which may be held in relation to the adult (Figure 5.2) and professional/organisation (Figure 5.3) if something goes wrong in a person's life.

Figure 5.2 Risk – concerns regarding the person

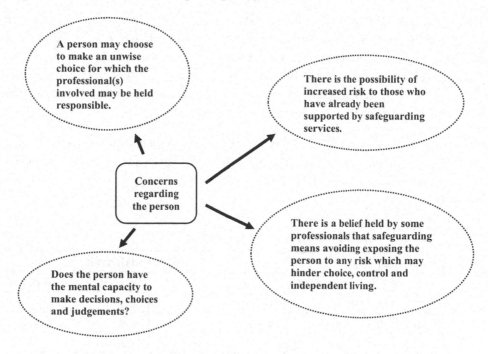

Figure 5.3 Risk – practitioner/organisational concerns

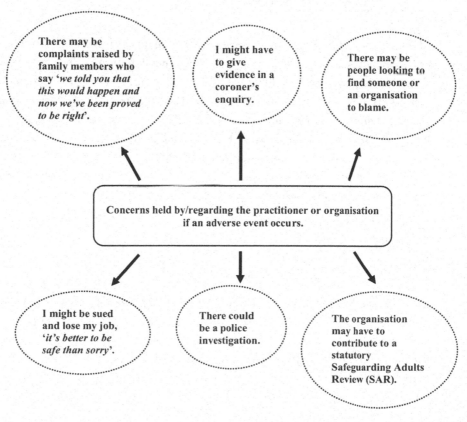

The conceptualisation of risk and risk management

There is no universally accepted definition of risk; however, it is often viewed in purely negative terms and is referred to solely in relation to a chance of an adverse or negative event occurring. Independence, choice and control are the principles, as practitioners, we strive to achieve with the adults we support; this can rest within a context of increasing fear of being held responsible if things go wrong, which can in itself lead to an increase in levels of risk aversion.

Studies by Taylor (2006) of a broad range of professionals involved in the long-term care of older adults showed that these practitioners conceptualised risk and its management according to six paradigms '*that seem to be in a state of reciprocal tension*' (Table 5.1).

Table 5.1 Concepts of risk – six paradigms

Six paradigms		Risk area
1.	Balancing benefits and harm	Choice and empowerment
2.	Identifying and meeting needs	Needs for services
3.	Minimising situational hazards	Health and safety
4.	Protecting the individual	Safeguarding
5.	Accounting for resources and priorities	Eligibility and resources
6.	Wariness of lurking conflicts	

There is a need for all practitioners involved with an adult to be able to differentiate between safeguarding, risk aversion and the crucial differences between real/actual risk and perceptions of risk. In his article *Stop Worrying About Risk*, Stephen Finlayson (2015) argues '*it is time to use ordinary language that creates ordinary responses – to stop worrying about risk – and start talking about our worries*'. In this piece of work, Finlayson discusses the increasing focus placed, in social care, on 'risk enablement', 'risk assessment' and 'risk management', and promotes a return to '*ordinary language and ordinary ways of doing things*'. He describes his own use of three simple questions, which may be a useful starting point for all practitioners:

» What are we worried about?

» How worried are we?

» What can we do to worry less?

An example described within *Stop Worrying About Risk* is a situation where the mother of a man with a learning disability is concerned about the risks associated with his choice to go out clubbing (and '*perhaps even wanting to get very drunk with friends*') – it is an interesting read for practitioners wishing to take their own thinking and practice further.

Practitioners should always work to ensure that all safeguarding interventions fully involve supporting the adult at risk to develop resilience and personal coping strategies, with the primary aim of empowering them to manage and mitigate risks for themselves. The now-famous statement made by the then Mr Justice Mumby (now Lord Justice Mumby) in the High Court of Justice (2007) is useful for us all to remember:

There is one final point to be made. The court, as I have said, is entitled to intervene to protect a vulnerable adult from the risk of future harm – the risk of future abuse or future exploitation – so long as there is a real possibility, rather than a merely fanciful risk, of such harm. But the court must adopt a pragmatic, common sense and robust approach to the identification, evaluation and management of perceived risk.

*A great judge once said, 'all life is an experiment,' adding that 'every year if not every day we have to wager our salvation upon some prophecy based upon imperfect knowledge' (see Holmes J in Abrams v United States (1919) 250 US 616 at pages 624, 630). The fact is that all life involves risk, and the young, the elderly and the vulnerable, are exposed to additional risks and to risks they are less well equipped than others to cope with. But just as wise parents resist the temptation to keep their children metaphorically wrapped up in cotton wool, so too we must avoid the temptation always to put the physical health and safety of the elderly and the vulnerable before everything else. Often it will be appropriate to do so, but not always. Physical health and safety can sometimes be bought at too high a price in happiness and emotional welfare. The emphasis must be on sensible risk appraisal, not striving to avoid all risk, whatever the price, but instead seeking a proper balance and being willing to tolerate manageable or acceptable risks as the price appropriately to be paid in order to achieve some other good – in particular to achieve the vital good of the elderly or vulnerable person's happiness. **What good is it making someone safer if it merely makes them miserable?***

 SnapShot on... **information-sharing**

In order to respond appropriately when abuse or neglect may be taking place, anyone in contact with the adult, whether in a voluntary or paid role, must understand their own role and responsibilities. They should also have access to practical and legal guidance, advice and support. This will include understanding local interagency policies and procedures, such as the Safeguarding Adults Board (SAB), Multi-agency Policy and Procedure, Multi-Agency Risk Assessment Conference (MARAC) and Multi-Agency Public Protection Arrangements (MAPPA). This *SnapShot...* has been updated to reflect the General Data Protection Regulations (Information Commissioner's Office, 2018).

» A MARAC is a meeting where information is shared on the highest risk domestic abuse cases between representatives of local police, health, child protection, housing practitioners, independent domestic violence advisers (IDVAs), probation and other specialists from the statutory and voluntary sectors.

» MAPPA are in place to ensure the successful management of violent and sexual offenders.

Clear organisational policies and procedures (or formally agreed and documented 'ways of working') should aim to give guidance on safeguarding prevention and early intervention procedures to follow if and when abuse or neglect has happened or is suspected.

Where there are safeguarding adult concerns, staff have a duty to share information. It is important to remember that in a number of Safeguarding Adults Reviews (SARs, previously known as Serious Case Reviews) ineffective information-sharing has been identified as a prominent factor. This was described as a factor within the SAR undertaken by the West Berkshire Safeguarding Adults Board (SAB) published in July 2016 regarding an adult named Mr I. This SAR report highlights particular issues in relation to the completion of case transfer processes and the updating of and access to key electronic care records across service disciplines; in this case a single point of access function and mental health services which took place during and following a period of agency restructure.

Staff should have a clear direction in what information should be recorded and in what format. A key consideration for any individual involved with suspected or actual abuse or neglect should be 'What information am I required to share and with whom, in order to manage the risk?'. We refer to this as the 'critical question wheel'; this is represented in graphic form as Figure 5.4.

Figure 5.4 The critical question wheel

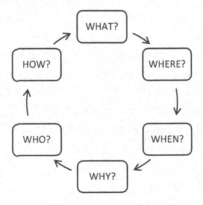

The Caldicott Principles

In December 1997, Dame Fiona Caldicott published a *Report on the Review of Patient-Identifiable Information*, which had been commissioned in 1997 by the Chief Medical Officer in England to address concerns surrounding the use of personal information within the NHS. This report contained a set of six principles which became known as the Caldicott Principles, after the report's author. In 2012, following a review, a seventh principle was added to the existing set. These seven principles are as follows.

1. **Justify the purpose(s).** Every single proposed use or transfer of patient identifiable information within or from an organisation should be clearly defined and scrutinised, with continuing uses regularly reviewed, by an appropriate guardian (called the Caldicott Guardian).

2. **Don't use patient identifiable information unless it is necessary.** Patient identifiable information items should not be included unless it is essential for the specified purpose(s) of that flow. The need for patients to be identified should be considered at each stage of satisfying the purpose(s).

3. **Use the minimum necessary patient-identifiable information.** Where use of patient identifiable information is considered to be essential, the inclusion of each individual item of information should be considered and justified so that the minimum amount of identifiable information is transferred or accessible as is necessary for a given function to be carried out.

4. **Access to patient identifiable information should be on a strict need-to-know basis.** Only those individuals who need access to patient identifiable information should have access to it, and they should only have access to the information items that they need to see. This may mean introducing access controls or splitting information flows where one information flow is used for several purposes.

5. **Everyone with access to patient identifiable information should be aware of their responsibilities.** Action should be taken to ensure that those handling patient identifiable information – both clinical and non-clinical staff – are made fully aware of their responsibilities and obligations to respect patient confidentiality.

6. **Understand and comply with the law.** Every use of patient identifiable information must be lawful. Someone in each organisation handling patient information should be responsible for ensuring that the organisation complies with legal requirements.

7. **The duty to share information can be as important as the duty to protect patient confidentiality.** Professionals should, in the patient's interest, share information within this framework. Official policies should support them doing so.

Seven golden rules in making safeguarding personal

1. The General Data Protection Regulations (Information Commissioner's Office, 2018) do not prevent or limit the sharing of information for the purpose of keeping people safe – they serve to ensure that personal information is shared appropriately (see Figure 5.5).

2. Be open and honest with the person (and/or their family or representative as appropriate) from the onset about *why, what, how* and *with whom* information will or could be shared. Seek their agreement unless it is unsafe or inappropriate to do so (clearly document all decisions confirming how they were arrived at).

3. Seek advice if you are in doubt – without disclosing the identity of the person where possible.

4. Information can be shared without consent to keep an individual at risk safe from neglect, physical, emotional or psychological harm or to protect their physical, emotional or psychological well-being. However, where possible, consent should be sought from the individual before information is shared.

5. Consider safety and well-being – base your information-sharing decisions on consideration of the safety and well-being of the person and others who may be affected by their actions (eg, carers).

6. Necessary, proportionate, relevant, accurate, timely, secure: ensure that the information you share is necessary for the purpose for which you are sharing it – these six factors are commonly referred to as the Caldicott Principles (further information is detailed above).

7. Keep a clear chronological record of **all** decisions, and the reasons they were made.

Figure 5.5 Flowchart of key aspects in information-sharing
(adapted from Guidance for Practitioners and Managers, HM Government, 2009)

You are asked to or wish to share information

Is there a clear and legitimate purpose for the sharing of this information? → NO

YES

Does the information identify a living person? → NO

YES

Is the information confidential? → NO

YES

Do you have consent? → YES

NO

Is there sufficient PUBLIC INTEREST to share the information? → YES

NOT SURE → SEEK ADVICE

YOU CAN SHARE

NO → DO NOT SHARE

SHARING the information:
- Identify how much to share
- Share FACT not opinion
- The right information to the right person
- Ensure security and safety of the information
- Inform the person that the information has been shared if they are not already aware and it will not create or increase risk of harm

RECORD the information sharing decision and your reasons in line with local practice

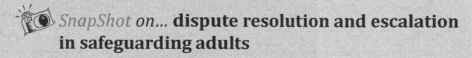

SnapShot on... **dispute resolution and escalation in safeguarding adults**

This *SnapShot* considers an approach towards the positive and proactive resolution of disputes or disagreements which can arise between practitioners involved in safeguarding adults cases. In cases where a dispute or disagreement is raised by the adult at risk, their representative or a carer, the agency's complaints policy should be followed, with the option of referral to the ombudsman when all other avenues to seek resolution are felt to have been exhausted.

Disputes and disagreements can arise for a multitude of reasons, many of which can be as a result of misunderstandings regarding the responsibilities held by partner agencies, and expectations of responses to be made. They can also arise as a result of the perceived limitations of organisational boundaries and common practice, particularly during a climate of resource pressure. At all times it is vital to keep in mind jointly held statutory duties, the priority being the safety and well-being of the adult concerned, and to maintain a positive, resolution-focused approach open to challenge and change.

The simple 'five-stage' resolution flowchart (Figure 5.6) is designed to support the achievement of resolution at the earliest opportunity and in a timely manner.

Figure 5.6 'Five-stage' resolution flowchart

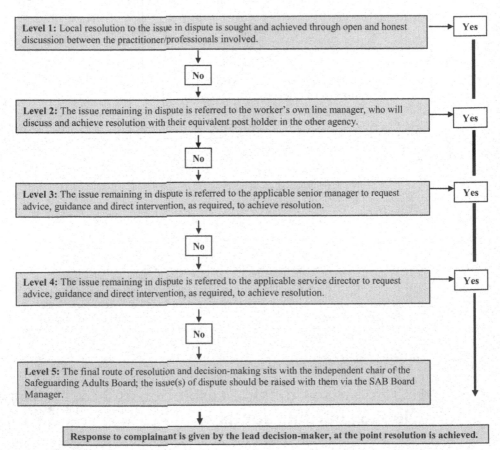

Level 1: Local resolution to the issue in dispute is sought and achieved through open and honest discussion between the practitioner/professionals involved. → Yes

No

Level 2: The issue remaining in dispute is referred to the worker's own line manager, who will discuss and achieve resolution with their equivalent post holder in the other agency. → Yes

No

Level 3: The issue remaining in dispute is referred to the applicable senior manager to request advice, guidance and direct intervention, as required, to achieve resolution. → Yes

No

Level 4: The issue remaining in dispute is referred to the applicable service director to request advice, guidance and direct intervention, as required, to achieve resolution. → Yes

No

Level 5: The final route of resolution and decision-making sits with the independent chair of the Safeguarding Adults Board; the issue(s) of dispute should be raised with them via the SAB Board Manager.

Response to complainant is given by the lead decision-maker, at the point resolution is achieved.

SnapShot on... the coroner and reports under Regulation 28

This *SnapShot* is designed to support practitioners in understanding the role of the coroner and Coroner's Office. Health and social care practitioners can be asked to provide the coroner with information in relation to the facts and circumstances surrounding their involvement with a person who has died. In work with adults with care and support needs, who have the mental capacity to make decisions about where, how and with whom they live, and who place themselves at severe risk of significant harm by the refusal of vital care and support services, which then leads to their death (eg, Mr I, West Berkshire SAR), the cause of their death will need to be established by the local coroner. This request will usually be made by the Coroner's Office and may be for a written report, copies of and/or original relevant documentation (this can include, for example, case records, Care Act needs assessments, Care and Support Plans, reviews), or attendance at an inquest.

Relevant legislation

» Coroners and Justice Act (2009).

» The Coroners (Investigations) Regulations (2013).

» The Coroners (Inquest) Rules (2013).

A coroner is a legally qualified and experienced solicitor or barrister; they fulfil an important role within the judicial system. When a death occurs, in particular circumstances (outlined below), it is the job of a coroner to establish the identity of the deceased person and the cause of their death.

If it appears that there is a risk of other deaths occurring in similar circumstances in the future, the coroner has the legal power and duty to write a report (or letter) which is sent to people or organisations who are in a position to act to reduce the risk. This is sometimes referred to as a Report under Regulation 28; this refers to the Coroners (Investigations) Regulations (2013). The recipient(s) of a Regulation 28 Report (or letter) must make a formal response within 56 days of receipt and detail what actions they will take; this is discussed further below.

When should the coroner be notified of a death?

When the deceased has:

(a) died a violent/unnatural death (including accident/ suicide);

(b) died, and the cause of death is unknown;

(c)   died while in custody or other form of state detention;

(d)   died as a result of medical treatment.

(NB: the list above is not exhaustive.)

Notifications to the coroner are usually made by a registered medical practitioner (doctor) or the police, but anyone who is concerned about the cause of death can contact their local Coroner's Office.

When should the coroner hold an inquest?

» To determine the medical cause of death.

» To investigate the circumstances of the death.

» To identify the existence of circumstances that, if action is not taken by a person or organisation, might lead to further deaths.

» To advance medical knowledge.

» To preserve the legal interest of the deceased's family or other interested parties.

Under Section 8(1) of the Coroners and Justice Act (2009) when the deceased:

(a)   has died a violent or unnatural death;

(b)   has died a sudden death of which the cause is unknown; or

(c)   has died in prison or in such a place or in such circumstances as to require an inquest under any other Act (Section 8(3) states this type of inquest must be held with a jury).

Types of hearings (open to the public)

Pre-inquest hearing

This is a hearing that the coroner may choose to hold in order to decide matters such as the scope and date of the inquest, the witnesses and evidence he/she plans to call and use. The coroner may also set out what else he/she needs to complete preparations for the inquest.

The inquest

This is a public hearing and fact-finding inquiry (with or without a jury) to establish who died, and how, when and where the death occurred.

NB: An inquest does not apportion blame regarding the death of a person – it seeks to establish the cause of death.

Possible verdicts

The following are possible cause of death verdicts/conclusions. However, in addition, the coroner can give what is known as a narrative verdict; this gives more detail about the reason for the verdict decision.

» Accident or misadventure.

» Alcohol/drug-related.

» Industrial disease.

» Lawful/unlawful killing (criminal standard of proof for the latter).

» Natural causes.

» Open verdict (where there is insufficient evidence for any other verdict).

» Road traffic collision.

» Stillbirth.

» Suicide (criminal standard of proof).

Regulation 28 – Coroner's Report

As noted above, the coroner has a legal power and duty to write a report following an inquest if it appears there is a risk of other deaths occurring in similar circumstances. This known as a 'Report under Regulation 28' or a Preventing Future Deaths Report; this power comes from Regulation 28 of the Coroners (Inquest) Regulations (2013).

Why it matters and what happens next

» When a death occurs in the health and social care sector, it is more important than ever to identify risks that might cause deaths in future and make sure action is taken immediately.

» The response must be provided to the coroner who made the request within 56 days of the date on which the report is sent.

» The response to a report must contain:

  » details of any action that has been taken or which it is proposed will be taken by the person giving the response or any other person whether in response to the report or otherwise and set out a timetable of the action taken or proposed to be taken; *or*

  » an explanation as to why no action is proposed.

» The coroner must send a copy of the report to the chief coroner and every interested person who in the coroner's opinion should receive it, including the appropriate Local Safeguarding Children's Board if the coroner believes the deceased was under the age of 18. The chief coroner may publish a copy of the report, or a summary of it, in such a manner as the chief coroner sees fit.

National learning themes from Regulation 28 coroner reports

» Poor record-keeping.

» Missed diagnosis.

» Not following NICE guidelines.

» Lack of continuity of care.

» Overprescribing of pain relief.

» Lack of GP appointments.

» No clinical record made.

» Poor clinical assessment.

Conclusion

This chapter has given an overview of some of the practice issues of relevance in the management of severe risk with adults who have care and support needs, but who refuse to engage with the planning or delivery of vital care and support. It has looked at aspects of the 'protection versus self-determination' debate in addressing the dilemma of managing the balance between protecting adults at risk against their right to self-determination as a serious challenge for all services. Following a risk management process does not and should not affect an individual's human rights but seeks to ensure that the relevant agencies exercise their duty of care in a robust manner that is reasonable and proportionate. The application of a clear and robust process should ensure all reasonable steps are taken to promote safety by a multi-agency group of professionals directly including, wherever and however possible, the adult at risk.

We have not been exhaustive in terms of either subject matter or detail but have planned to give a flavour and to spark interest in what we find is a demanding, challenging, but highly rewarding area of practice. Positive outcomes can be achieved when respectful professional curiosity, interest and a strong commitment to social justice and human rights are held at the forefront of our work. We strongly encourage all practitioners to undertake further research in order to build their practice toolkit of resources which are of key importance in this ever-evolving and complex area of their work; particularly in the use of published Safeguarding Adults Reviews as a source for continued professional awareness and development in the achievement of MSP and evidence-based practice. A selection of resources is included below.

Taking it further

References

Caldicott, F (1997) *The Caldicott Committee: Report on the Review of Patient-Identifiable Information*. London: Department of Health. [online] Available at: http://static.ukcgc.uk/docs/caldicott1.pdf (accessed 21 September 2020).

Court of Appeal (2018) *Before: Lord Justice Baker. Between: A Local Authority and BF*. [online] Available at: www.bailii.org/ew/cases/EWCA/Civ/2018/2962.pdf (accessed 21 September 2020).

Department of Health (2018) *Care and Support Statutory Guidance*. [online] Available at: www.gov.uk/government/publications/care-act-statutory-guidance/care-and-support-statutory-guidance (accessed 21 September 2020).

Finlayson, S (2015) *Stop Worrying About Risk*. Sheffield: Centre for Welfare Reform. [online] Available at: www.centreforwelfarereform.org/library/by-az/stop-worrying-about-risk.html (accessed 21 September 2020).

Heighton, A (2017) *Driving and Restraining Forces to Consider When Utilising a Conceptual Risks and Strengths Assessment Model: A Human Perspective*. Given as a presentation (unpublished).

High Court of Justice (2007) *Local Authority X v MM and KM*. [online] Available at: www.bailii.org/ew/cases/EWHC/Fam/2007/2003.html (accessed 21 September 2020).

HM Government (1998) *Human Rights Act 1998*. Norwich: The Stationery Office. [online] Available at: www.legislation.gov.uk/ukpga/1998/42/contents (accessed 21 September 2020).

HM Government (2009) Coroners and Justice Act 2009. Norwich: The Stationery Office. [online] Available at: www.legislation.gov.uk/ukpga/2009/25/pdfs/ukpga_20090025_en.pdf (accessed 21 September 2020).

HM Government (2013a) The Coroners (Investigations) Regulations 2013. Norwich: The Stationery Office. [online] Available at: www.legislation.gov.uk/uksi/2013/1629/pdfs/uksi_20131629_en.pdf (accessed 21 September 2020).

HM Government (2013b) The Coroners (Inquests) Rules 2013. Norwich: The Stationery Office. [online] Available at: www.legislation.gov.uk/uksi/2013/1616/pdfs/uksi_20131616_en.pdf (accessed 21 September 2020).

House of Lords (1990) *Re F (Sterilisation: Mental Patient)*. [online] Available at: www.bailii.org/uk/cases/UKHL/1991/1.html (accessed 21 September 2020).

Information Commissioner's Office (2018) *Guide to the General Data Protection Regulations*. London: HM Government. [online] Available at: https://assets.publishing.service.gov.uk/government/uploads/system/uploads/attachment_data/file/711097/guide-to-the-general-data-protection-regulation-gdpr-1-0.pdf (accessed 21 September 2020).

Taylor, B (2006) Risk Management Paradigms in Health and Social Services for Professional Decision Making on the Long-term Care of Older People. *British Journal of Social Work*, 36(8): 1411–29.

West Berkshire Safeguarding Adults Board (2016) *Safeguarding Adults Review: Mr I*. [online] Available at: www.sabberkshirewest.co.uk/media/1202/sar-mr-i-final-report-2016v4.pdf (accessed 21 September 2020).

Publications

Faulkner, A and Sweeney, A (2011) *Report 41: Prevention in Adult Safeguarding*. Social Care Institute for Excellence (SCIE). [online] Available at: www.scie.org.uk/publications/reports/report41/ (accessed 21 September 2020).

Gigerenzer, G (2014) *Risk Savvy: How to Make Good Decisions*. New York: Penguin.

HM Government (2009) *Information Sharing: Guidance for Practitioners and Managers*. Department for Children, Schools and Families Publications. Nottingham, UK. Archived 26/03/2015. [online] Available at: https://www.gov.uk/government/publications/information-sharing-for-practitioners-and-managers (accessed 25 October 2020).

Taylor, B, Kellick, C and McGlade, A (2015) *Understanding and Using Research in Social Work*. London: Learning Matters.

Department of Health, ADASS and LGA (2018 [2014]) *Gaining Access to an Adult Suspected to be at Risk of Neglect or Abuse: A Guide for Social Workers and their Managers in England*. London: Social Care Institute for Excellence (SCIE). [online] Available at: www.scie.org.uk/files/safeguarding/adults/practice/gaining-access/gaining-access-to-an-adult-at-risk.pdf (accessed 21 September 2020).

Websites

Iriss on Risk: www.iriss.org.uk/resources/irisson/risk (accessed 21 September 2020).

NHS: Coroner's Regulation 28 Reports: www.wwl.nhs.uk/about_us/coroners_regulation_28_reports.aspx (accessed 21 September 2020).

Courts and Tribunals Judiciary: www.judiciary.gov.uk (accessed 21 September 2020).

Introduction

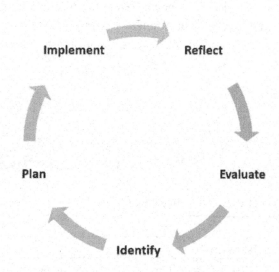

The critical review and evaluation of practice is vital to inform and direct the ongoing improvement of the experiences of the people who use services (and their carers) and as an aid to practitioners in their continued professional development. In order to promote and sustain effective outcome-focused and reflective practice, the authors have designed and used the following example tool formats included in this chapter. These simple tools are designed to be used by an individual practitioner to review their own casework and also as a framework for peer evaluation and reflective casework discussion.

The *SnapShots on...* included in this chapter are:

» Self/Peer Case Recording Review.

» MSP Practitioner 'Reflective Practice' Resource.

The prompts included within the Self/Peer Case Recording Review Tool (Table 6.1) are framed by the registration requirements of both the Nursing and Midwifery Council (NMC) and Social Work England (SWE), and they reflect statutory social work interventions contained within the Care Act (2014) and *Care and Support Statutory Guidance* (Department of Health, 2018). The individual elements described in the tool do not conflict with or replace regulatory responsibilities or professional requirements applicable to specific settings, more the tool can be used flexibly as a standalone 'short checking' resource or be amended by the practitioner to meet their individual needs. The measures included are three simple elements (Yes, No, Not Applicable), within which the practitioner – or if used as a 'peer to peer' resource their colleague reviewer – can add their own sources of evidence or comment as aids to future practice development as they wish.

The MSP Practitioner 'Reflective Practice' Resource (Table 6.2) is designed to give practitioners a simple framework for the critical evaluation of their own practice (including Safeguarding Enquiries) using the 'Six MSP Principles'. This framework can be adapted to reflect wider practice issues and be used as an aid to continued professional development by individual workers, peers, teams and services as a means to identify, plan and implement practice/service improvements to achieve real and meaningful outcomes for the people directly involved through what can be an extremely difficult, distressing and confusing time for them.

Practice matters

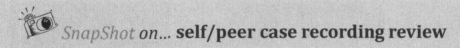 *SnapShot on...* **self/peer case recording review**

Table 6.1 Self/Peer Case Recording Review Tool

Element	Yes	No	N/A
Care Act Needs Assessment			
The Care Act (2014) Needs Assessment is proportionate to the presenting situation and circumstances of the person, is compliant with statutory duties and promotes their strengths, autonomy and human rights.			
Required planning with the person of the date, time and location of the Needs Assessment visit (or visits) has been completed and they have identified who they would like to be present; this is documented.			
The person has been supported with their preferred/required form of communication (eg, interpreter, translator, etc).			
The mental capacity of the person has been considered and the support of independent advocacy has been offered as applicable – in line with the statutory requirements of the Mental Capacity Act (2005) and/or Care Act (2014) and all other applicable legislation.			
In cases where the Mental Capacity Act (2005) applies, all decisions and time-specific Mental Capacity Assessments are fully completed, and are, as applicable accompanied by documented best interests decisions.			
The safety and well-being of the person (and, as applicable, their carer) has been considered in line with the Care Act (2014) and the Human Rights Act (1998). Risk and safety strategies are explored with the person – all plans agreed are proportionate.			

Element	Yes	No	N/A
All identified Safeguarding Concerns have been clearly documented, with actions taken in line with the Care Act (2014) legal requirements and operational procedure.			
The person's voice is clearly reflected and has been listened to, and all strengths, natural assets and individual resources to meet needs and those of members of their significant network have been explored.			
Where a carer is involved, an assessment of their needs (either joint or individual) has been offered; this is documented			
Multi-agency involvement is clearly documented including consideration of the person's eligibility for NHS Continuing Health Care funding (including Funded Nursing Care Contribution as applicable).			
A direct payment has been considered and discussed with the person as applicable, with accessible information explained and given to them.			
All financial costs (based upon their indicative personal budget) have been discussed with, understood and agreed by the person (or representative).			
All decision-making processes are clearly and concisely documented – giving reasons for how and why a decision has been reached, highlighting the personal outcome(s) to be achieved, any relevant challenges, differing views, tensions or areas of dispute (this may include aspects of discrimination which affect/impact the person).			
Information in an accessible format of how to make a complaint or compliment has been given.			

Element	Yes	No	N/A
Care and support planning (*or* support planning)			
The Care and Support Plan or Support Plan (the Plan) details how the person wishes to stay well, healthy and safe by confirming their goals, outcomes, eligible needs and how they will be met within the indicative budget.			
A strengths-based approach has been taken in the Plan which identifies and mitigates any power imbalances or potential areas of discrimination with the person, by the adoption of a creative, positive and respectfully critically curious approach, utilising all natural and community resources available to the person.			
Assistive technologies have been considered as contributions to meeting the person's defined outcomes and to promote their autonomy and independence.			
The person has been given the opportunity to design their own Plan in their chosen format.			
Evidence of how known risks will be positively managed is recorded.			

Element	Yes	No	N/A
Confirmation of how the Plan will be sustained and contingency planning completed (What if ...) in the event of deterioration and/or fluctuations in the person's strengths or abilities or those of their carer – in line with the Human Rights Act (1998) and, as applicable, Mental Capacity Act (2005), Mental Health Act (1983), Care Act (2014), and all other legislative requirements and professional responsibilities.			
Evidence that, where applicable, the person has been involved, and has directed how the personal budget or direct payment will be spent.			
Evidence of clear communication with the person (in line with their needs) of any financial cost to them as their contribution to their Plan.			
The person has received and agreed a copy of their Plan, which details how their eligible needs (including where applicable non-eligible needs) will be met and when it will be reviewed.			

Element	Yes	No	N/A
Review of Care and Support Plans (*or* Support Plans)			
Required planning with the person of the date, time and location of the review has been completed and they have identified who they would like to be present; this is documented and proportionate to the individual situation.			
The person has been supported with their preferred/required form of communication (eg, interpreter, translator, etc).			
Where the person is in receipt of commissioned services (eg, domiciliary care or in a care home setting), arrangements have also been agreed with the provider of that service.			
Where the person is in receipt of a direct payment it has been established that all spending is in line with and continues to meet agreed goals/outcomes, with no known concerns.			
Evidence that the original outcomes have been analysed and assessed with the person against their current needs with the Plan updated as required with the person clearly retaining decision-making control as applicable.			
All changes to the Plan are clearly documented and communicated to the person and all relevant parties. These may include, for example: • updates to the outcomes to be achieved; • adjustments to the Plan.			
The person has received a copy of their reviewed and updated Plan which details how their eligible needs (including where applicable non-eligible needs) will be met.			
There is a clear timescale for the completion of the next review, which has been agreed with the person and is proportionate to the outcomes confirmed.			

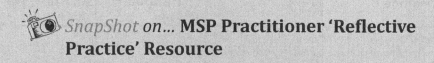

SnapShot on... **MSP Practitioner 'Reflective Practice' Resource**

Table 6.2 Practitioner 'Reflective Practice' Resource

Empowerment	I have achieved this by	I can improve this by
I have respected and responded to the personal and protected characteristics of the adult at risk, using this to inform all enquiry, planning and decision-making processes.		
I have considered the adult at risk's advocacy and/or support needs in order that they are able to fully participate in the Safeguarding Enquiry and made this available as applicable.		
I have explained the Safeguarding Enquiry process in an appropriate and accessible format to the adult at risk and/or their advocate.		
I have recorded and responded to the adult at risk's voice and their own words to confirm what safe means to them, their desired outcome and how it will be achieved.		
I have made sure that I have invited the adult at risk and/or their advocate to all relevant planning meetings, and where they haven't been able to attend, I have communicated clearly, accurately and concisely.		
I have gathered the views of the adult at risk and/or their advocate about their experience of the Safeguarding Enquiry process (where appropriate); this includes providing information resources in an appropriate and accessible format about how to submit a complaint and/or compliment.		
Prevention	**I have achieved this by**	**I can improve this by**
I have explained what abuse and neglect are, and how to report any concerns to the adult at risk and/or their advocate.		
I have respected the human rights of the adult at risk in assessment and risk management planning and, where applicable, have incorporated longer-term positive risk-taking strategies to meet person-centred outcomes.		

Prevention	I have achieved this by	I can improve this by
I have confirmed the conclusion of the Safe-guarding Enquiry on the balance of probability, and have identified, as applicable, actions taken and planned to mitigate the risk of abuse or neglect reoccurring to the adult at risk or other adults at risk.		
I have identified and shared learning from this Safeguarding Enquiry with my organisation to aid future development.		
Proportionality	**I have achieved this by**	**I can improve this by**
I have clearly documented the decision-making process to undertake a Safeguarding Enquiry; it is proportionate to the concern raised and is the least intrusive approach possible to meet statutory duties.		
I have evidenced the 'well-being principle' in all of my practice and decision-making.		
I have recorded all strategy meetings and discussions; the records specify actions to be taken, why, by whom and within what timescales.		
I have undertaken and completed the Safe-guarding Enquiry within a timescale that is proportionate to the complexity of risk identified and have avoided unnecessary delay.		
Protection	**I have achieved this by**	**I can improve this by**
I have documented all immediate actions taken to ensure the safety of the adult at risk, and that of other adults at risk or children also involved.		
I assessed the adult at risk's mental capacity in line with the requirements of the Mental Capacity Act (2005); this is clearly documented with best interests decision-making as app-licable.		
I have considered and appropriately addressed the mental capacity of the alleged source of harm where they are an adult at risk, and there were concerns that they may lack mental capacity in relation to the concern raised.		
I have clearly documented all protective ac-tions declined by the adult at risk, particularly in relation to their disengagement with the Safeguarding Enquiry and/or protection plan.		

Protection	I have achieved this by	I can improve this by
I have concluded the Safeguarding Enquiry within the required timescale; where this has not been achieved, I have clearly documented the reasons why.		

Partnership	I have achieved this by	I can improve this by
I have worked in partnership with the adult at risk and/or their advocate throughout the Safeguarding Enquiry process.		
I have sought the involvement of partner agencies at the time it was needed.		
I have clearly documented all communications and information-sharing between parties involved in the Safeguarding Enquiry.		
I have shared information in a timely manner in line with national standards and legal requirements.		
I have given feedback to all parties involved in the Safeguarding Enquiry appropriately and in line with applicable legal requirements.		
I have clearly documented all disputes or disagreements that arose and dealt with these positively in the best interests of the adult at risk; where these arose between practitioners the applicable Escalation Procedure was used and/or where the adult at risk disengaged with the Safeguarding Enquiry the Safeguarding Risk Management Protocol was followed.		
I have made referrals to other agencies/ systems as applicable (this could include, eg, MARAC, PREVENT, CQC).		

Accountability	I have achieved this by	I can improve this by
I have sought and engaged in practice supervision relating to the Safeguarding Enquiry appropriately.		
I have ensured management oversight and authorisations as applicable.		
I have clearly explained and documented the reason(s) for all delays.		
I have clearly explained and documented the reason(s) why the adult at risk's desired outcome(s) were not achieved, as applicable.		

Accountability	I have achieved this by	I can improve this by
I have created and implemented a protection plan with the adult at risk, and/or their advocate; all planned actions detail what action is to be taken, why, when and by whom.		
The adult at risk and/or their advocate has received a copy of the Safeguarding Enquiry Outcome Report, including cases where the adult at risk has ceased their involvement.		

Taking it further

Department of Health and Social Care (2019) *Strengths-based Approach: Practice Framework and Practice Handbook*. [online] Available at: https://assets.publishing.service.gov.uk/government/uploads/system/uploads/attachment_data/file/778134/stengths-based-approach-practice-framework-and-handbook.pdf (accessed 21 September 2020).

Index

abuse, 69
  as adverse childhood experience (ACE), 79
  case scenario CD, 28, 73, 101
  case scenario JA, 72, 97
  and coercive behaviour, 42, 44
  definition of, 42
  Domestic Abuse Bill (2020), 44
  domestic abuse practitioner toolkit, 46
  gendered nature of, 45–6
  identifying and referring, 82
  and information sharing, 123, 124
  and mate crime, 52–3
  and multi-agency working, 108, 118
  as part of three-stage test, 7, 9, 110, 113
  protection from, 105, 106, 107, 109, 110
  reaction to, 78
  relationship with illegal drugs, 51
  risk of, 89, 90, 122
  serious abuse and death, 111
  and 'toxic trio', 81
  see also domestic violence and abuse
accountability principle (*Care and Support Statutory Guidance*), 7
active listening, 18–20, 61
adolescence, documenting in story board, 24, 29
Adult Attachment Interview (AAI), 77
adult family violence (AFV), 81
adulthood, documenting in story board, 25, 29
adverse childhood experiences (ACEs), 70, 73, 79, 82–5
  ACEs pyramid, 85
  factors relating to child, 83
  factors relating to parent/household, 84
  personal thoughts and feelings, 86
advocacy, 15, 35–7
Ainsworth, M D, 75, 76, 78
Amnesty International UK, 45, 46
anti-discriminatory practice (ADP), 15
anti-oppressive practice (AOP), 15
assessment of need, 14
Association of Directors of Adult Social Services (ADASS), 7
attachment and attachment styles, 70, 74–80
  case scenarios CD, 73
  case scenario JA, 72
Autism spectrum disorder, 9, 25, 76

Baker, N, 36
best interests decision-making, 39–40
Black and Minority Ethnic (BME)/Black, Asian and Minority Ethnic (BAME) communities
  and advocacy, 36–7

  and diversity of need, 36
  terminology, 37
Black, use of terminology, 37
Blackburn, S, 46
body language, 19–20
Bowlby, J, 6, 74–6, 77
Boy Who Was Raised as a Dog, The (book), 78
Bretherton, I, 76
British Association of Social Workers (BASW), 21
British Journal of Social Work, 8

Caldicott Principles, 125–6
Caldicott, F, 125
Care and Support Plans, 101, 102
  principles in, 93–5
Care and Support Statutory Guidance (Department of Health, 2018), 8, 11, 135
  eligible and non-eligible needs, 31–3
  multi-agency working, 109
  three-stage test, 9, 113
Care Act (2014), 7, 9, 14, 51, 135
  advocacy, 35–7
  eligible and non-eligible needs, 31–3
  and protection planning, 89
  Safeguarding Adult Boards (SABs), 110–11
  strengths-based approach, 11
  and well-being, 104–7
care management, 8, 14
case scenarios (CD)
  advocacy, 37
  background, 9–10
  Care and Support Plan review, 101
  eligible needs, 34
  initial approach and story board, 27–9
  mental capacity, 41
  protection planning, 54, 102
  risks and strengths assessment, 72
case scenarios (JA)
  advocacy, 37
  background, 9
  eligible needs, 34
  initial approach and story board, 23–6
  mental capacity, 41
  protection planning, 54, 96
  risks and strengths assessment, 71
Centers for Disease Control and Prevention (CDC), 83
change, resistance to, 116
chronology, use of, 54–6, 92
clarification skills, 20
coercive control, 41–3, 120
  collating evidence of, 48–9
cognitive fluctuation, 65, 66